Pulmonary Disease in the Aging Patient

Editors

SIDNEY S. BRAMAN
GWEN S. SKLOOT

CLINICS IN GERIATRIC MEDICINE

www.geriatric.theclinics.com

November 2017 • Volume 33 • Number 4

ELSEVIER

1600 John F. Kennedy Boulevard • Suite 1800 • Philadelphia, Pennsylvania, 19103-2899

http://www.theclinics.com

CLINICS IN GERIATRIC MEDICINE Volume 33, Number 4
November 2017 ISSN 0749–0690, ISBN-13: 978-0-323-54879-3

Editor: Jessica McCool
Developmental Editor: Colleen Dietzler

Clinics in Geriatric Medicine (ISSN 0749-0690) is published quarterly by Elsevier Inc., 360 Park Avenue South, New York, NY 10010-1710. Months of issue are February, May, August, and November. Business and Editorial Offices: 1600 John F. Kennedy Blvd., Suite 1800, Philadelphia, PA 191023-2899. Periodicals postage paid at New York, NY, and additional mailing offices. Subscription prices are $273.00 per year (US individuals), $590.00 per year (US institutions), $100.00 per year (US student/resident), $381.00 per year (Canadian individuals), $748.00 per year (Canadian institutions), $195.00 per year (Canadian student/resident), $402.00 per year (international individuals), $748.00 per year (international institutions), and $195.00 per year (international student/resident). Foreign air speed delivery is included in all *Clinics* subscription prices. All prices are subject to change without notice. POSTMASTER: Send address changes to *Clinics in Geriatric Medicine*, Elsevier Health Sciences Division, Subscription Customer Service, 3251 Riverport Lane, Maryland Heights, MO 63043. **Telephone: 1-800-654-2452 (U.S. and Canada); 314-447-8871 (outside U.S. and Canada). Fax: 314-447-8029. E-mail:** journalscustomerservice-usa@elsevier.com **(for print support) or** journalsonlinesupport-usa@elsevier.com **(for online support).**

Reprints. For copies of 100 or more, of articles in this publication, please contact the Commercial Reprints Department, Elsevier Inc., 360 Park Avenue South, New York, New York 10010-1710. Tel.: 212-633-3874; Fax: 212-633-3820, E-mail: reprints@elsevier.com.

Clinics in Geriatric Medicine is covered in *MEDLINE/PubMed (Index Medicus), EMBASE/Excerpta Medica, Current Contents/Clinical Medicine (CC/CM),* and the *Cumulative Index to Nursing & Allied Health Literature.*

Contributors

EDITORS

SIDNEY S. BRAMAN, MD, FCCP
Professor, Department of Medicine, Division of Pulmonary, Critical Care and Sleep Medicine, Icahn School of Medicine at Mount Sinai, New York, New York, USA

GWEN S. SKLOOT, MD, FACCP
Professor, Department of Medicine, Division of Pulmonary, Critical Care and Sleep Medicine, Icahn School of Medicine at Mount Sinai, New York, New York, USA

AUTHORS

KORI ASCHER, DO
Pulmonary Critical Care Fellow, Department of Medicine, Division of Pulmonary, Allergy, Critical Care and Sleep Medicine, University of Miami Miller School of Medicine, Miami, Florida, USA

JULIE A. BARTA, MD
Division of Pulmonary and Critical Care Medicine, Sidney Kimmel Medical College, Thomas Jefferson University, Philadelphia, Pennsylvania, USA

DEVIN M. BOE, BA
Division of GI, Trauma and Endocrine Surgery, Department of Surgery, Mucosal Inflammation Program, Graduate Program in Immunology, University of Colorado Anschutz Medical Campus, Aurora, Colorado, USA

LISBETH A. BOULE, PhD
Division of GI, Trauma and Endocrine Surgery, Department of Surgery, Mucosal Inflammation Program, IMAGE, University of Colorado Anschutz Medical Campus, Aurora, Colorado, USA

SIDNEY S. BRAMAN, MD, FCCP
Professor, Department of Medicine, Division of Pulmonary, Critical Care and Sleep Medicine, Icahn School of Medicine at Mount Sinai, New York, New York, USA

FELIPE CORTOPASSI, PT, RPFT, MBA
Pulmonary Department, Hospital Universitario Pedro Ernesto, Rio de Janeiro State University, Rio de Janeiro, Rio de Janeiro, Brazil

BRENDA J. CURTIS, PhD
Division of GI, Trauma and Endocrine Surgery, Department of Surgery, Mucosal Inflammation Program, IMAGE, University of Colorado Anschutz Medical Campus, Aurora, Colorado, USA

SHARON J. ELLIOT, PhD
Research Professor, DeWitt Daughtry Family Department of Surgery, University of Miami Miller School of Medicine, Miami, Florida, USA

STEVEN H. FEINSILVER, MD
Professor, Department of Medicine, Hofstra Northwell School of Medicine, Director, Center for Sleep Medicine, Lenox Hill Hospital, New York, New York, USA

MARILYN K. GLASSBERG, MD
Professor, Department of Medicine, Division of Pulmonary, Allergy, Critical Care and Sleep Medicine, Professor, DeWitt Daughtry Family Department of Surgery, Department of Pediatrics, Division of Pediatric Pulmonology, University of Miami Miller School of Medicine, Miami, Florida, USA

PUNCHO GURUNG, MD
Pulmonary-Critical Care Medicine Division, Baystate Medical Center, Springfield, Massachusetts, USA; Assistant Professor, Department of Medicine, Tufts University School of Medicine, Boston, Massachusetts, USA

ADAM B. HERNANDEZ, MD
Sleep Disorders Centers of the Mid-Atlantic, Glen Burnie, Maryland, USA

ELIZABETH J. KOVACS, PhD
Professor, Director of Burn Research, Director, Alcohol Research Program, Division of GI, Trauma and Endocrine Surgery, Department of Surgery, Mucosal Inflammation Program, GILIIP (GI, Liver and Innate Immunity Program), Graduate Program in Immunology, IMAGE, University of Colorado Anschutz Medical Campus, Aurora, Colorado, USA

DONALD A. MAHLER, MD
Emeritus Professor, Department of Medicine, Geisel School of Medicine at Dartmouth, Hanover, New Hampshire, USA; Director of Respiratory Services, Director of Clinical Resource Center of the Alpha-1 Foundation, Valley Regional Healthcare, Claremont, New Hampshire, USA

VICTOR PINTO-PLATA, MD
Pulmonary-Critical Care Medicine Division, Baystate Medical Center, Springfield, Massachusetts, USA; Assistant Professor, Department of Medicine, Tufts University School of Medicine, Boston, Massachusetts, USA

HOOMAN POOR, MD
Assistant Professor, Department of Medicine, Division of Pulmonary, Critical Care, and Sleep Medicine, Icahn School of Medicine at Mount Sinai, New York, New York, USA

GUSTAVO A. RUBIO, MD
Resident, DeWitt Daughtry Family Department of Surgery, University of Miami Miller School of Medicine, Miami, Florida, USA

NICOLA SCICHILONE, MD, PhD
Professor of Respiratory Diseases, Dipartimento di Biomedicina e Medicina Specialistica, Sezione di Pneumologia, University of Palermo, Palermo, Italy

GWEN S. SKLOOT, MD, FACCP
Professor, Department of Medicine, Division of Pulmonary, Critical Care and Sleep Medicine, Icahn School of Medicine at Mount Sinai, New York, New York, USA

MICHAEL UNGER, MD
Division of Pulmonary and Critical Care Medicine, Sidney Kimmel Medical College, Thomas Jefferson University, Philadelphia, Pennsylvania, USA

CARLOS A. VAZ FRAGOSO, MD
Department of Internal Medicine, Clinical Epidemiology Research Center, U.S. Department of Veterans Affairs, West Haven, Connecticut, USA; Department of Internal Medicine, Yale School of Medicine, New Haven, Connecticut, USA

RALPH G. ZINNER, MD
Department of Medical Oncology, Sidney Kimmel Medical College, Thomas Jefferson University, Philadelphia, Pennsylvania, USA

Contents

> Growth of the segment of the population older than 65 years has led to intensified interest in understanding the biology of aging. This article is focused on age-related alterations in lung structure that produce predictable changes in physiologic function, both at rest and during exercise. Increased insight into the physiology of the healthy aging lung should ultimately lead to improved methods of lung function assessment in the elderly (defined as those older than 65 years) as well as better understanding of the manifestations and possibly even the treatment of geriatric lung disease.

> With the coming of the "silver tsunami," expanding the knowledge about how various intrinsic and extrinsic factors affect the immune system in the elderly is timely and of immediate clinical need. The global population is increasing in age. By 2030, more than 20% of the population of the United States will be older than 65. This article focuses on how advanced age alters the immune systems and how this, in turn, modulates the ability of the aging lung to deal with infectious challenges from the outside world and from within the host.

> Natural lung aging is characterized by molecular and cellular changes in multiple lung cell populations. These changes include shorter telomeres, increased expression of cellular senescence markers, increased DNA damage, oxidative stress, apoptosis, and stem cell exhaustion. Aging, combined with the loss of protective repair processes, correlates with the development and incidence of chronic respiratory diseases, including idiopathic pulmonary fibrosis and chronic obstructive pulmonary disease. Ultimately, it is the interplay of age-related changes in biology and the subsequent responses to environmental exposures that largely define the physiology and clinical course of the aging lung.

> Older persons frequently report respiratory risk factors and symptoms and have a high prevalence of symptomatic lung disease, most commonly

obstructive airway disease, interstitial lung disease, and lung cancer. Notably, coexisting nonrespiratory risk factors are also prevalent and may misidentify or modify respiratory diagnoses and their clinical course.

Dyspnea is due to an imbalance between the *demand to breathe* and the *ability to breathe*. The prevalence is ~30% for those 65 years or older with walking on a level surface or up an incline. Dyspnea is a strong predictor of mortality in elderly individuals. Anemia, cardiovascular disease, deconditioning, psychological disorders, and respiratory diseases are common causes of dyspnea. Initial treatments to relieve breathing discomfort should be directed toward improving the pathophysiology of the underlying disease. Simple and inexpensive strategies to relieve dyspnea are available. This article provides an update on the evaluation of chronic dyspnea in elderly individuals.

The older population has seen the greatest increase in the prevalence of current asthma in recent years. Asthma may begin at any age and when it occurs at an advanced as opposed to a young age, it is often nonatopic, severe, and unremitting. Unfortunately, geriatric-specific guidelines are not available for the diagnosis and treatment of asthma. However, with objective monitoring, avoidance of asthma triggers, appropriate pharmacotherapy, and patient education, the disease can be managed successfully.

Chronic obstructive pulmonary disease (COPD) is prevalent in the elderly population, with high impact on quality of life, morbidity, and mortality. The diagnosis is usually made based on symptoms and spirometry values that support the presence of airflow obstruction. However, the condition is frequently underdiagnosed. COPD is associated with premature aging and several other medical conditions that can partially explain its underdiagnosis and management. There are several pharmacologic and nonpharmacologic interventions proven to be effective in ameliorating the symptoms of COPD. Appropriate drug delivery and reduction of side effects is also pivotal in the management of patients with COPD.

Pulmonary hypertension is a pathologic hemodynamic condition defined by a mean pulmonary arterial pressure of 25 mm Hg or greater at rest. Because of age-associated stiffening of the heart and the pulmonary vasculature and the higher prevalence in the elderly of comorbidities associated with the development of pulmonary hypertension, it is an increasingly common finding in this patient population. A right heart catheterization is necessary for the diagnosis and characterization of pulmonary hypertension. The general management is to treat the underlying conditions responsible for the development of the disorder. Pulmonary vasodilators are indicated in patients with pulmonary arterial hypertension.

CLINICS IN GERIATRIC MEDICINE

THE CLINICS ARE AVAILABLE ONLINE!
Access your subscription at:
www.theclinics.com

Preface
Pulmonary Disease in the Aging Patient

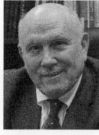 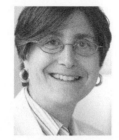

Sidney S. Braman, MD, FCCP Gwen S. Skloot, MD, FACCP
Editors

Every 24 hours, 10,000 liters of air are breathed into the lungs. This means that on a daily basis, we are exposed to large amounts of suspended particulate matter, noxious gasses, aeroallergens, and microbes that have the potential to cause disease. Changes in the immune system of elderly individuals (>65 years) coupled with aging-related physiologic changes of the respiratory system make this population more vulnerable to these dangers from the environment. While the protective mechanisms of the lungs are highly effective on most days, on very high pollution days, there are more hospital admissions in the elderly population for conditions such as pneumonia, chronic obstructive pulmonary disease (COPD) and asthma exacerbations, and coronary artery disease. What we do not know is the cumulative effect of these pollutants over a lifetime and how the lungs of the elderly are affected by this constant assault. This issue of the *Clinics in Geriatric Medicine* will explore the changes of aging and how risk factors for lung disease affect this vulnerable population. Specific lung diseases that are prevalent in the elderly, such as asthma, COPD, lung cancer, sleep-disordered breathing, and pulmonary hypertension, are discussed. In addition, as other nonrespiratory comorbidities are so common in elderly individuals and can affect the diagnosis and treatment of various lung diseases, a multidimensional approach to the older patient with respiratory conditions is presented.

Sidney S. Braman, MD, FCCP
Department of Medicine
Division of Medicine, Pulmonary, Critical Care, and Sleep Medicine
Icahn School of Medicine at Mount Sinai
One Gustav L. Levy Place, Box 1232, New York, NY 10029-6574, USA

Clin Geriatr Med 33 (2017) xi–xii
http://dx.doi.org/10.1016/j.cger.2017.08.001
0749-0690/17/© 2017 Published by Elsevier Inc.
geriatric.theclinics.com

Gwen S. Skloot, MD, FACCP
Department of Medicine
Division of Medicine, Pulmonary, Critical Care, and Sleep Medicine
Icahn School of Medicine at Mount Sinai
One Gustav L. Levy Place, Box 1232, New York, NY 10029-6574, USA

E-mail addresses:
sidney.braman@mssm.edu (S.S. Braman)
gwen.skloot@mssm.edu (G.S. Skloot)

The Effects of Aging on Lung Structure and Function

Gwen S. Skloot, MD, FACCP

KEYWORDS

• Aging • Lung structure • Lung function • Respiratory mechanics • Gas exchange

KEY POINTS

- The aging process alters the intrinsic structure of the lung as well as of the supportive extrapulmonary structures (ie, chest wall, spine, and respiratory muscles).
- These structural changes lead to unfavorable respiratory mechanics associated with decreased expiratory flows, increased air trapping and closing volume, and decreased gas exchange.
- The changes in lung structure and resting lung function impact exercise physiology in the elderly.
- Lung function testing in the elderly is generally a helpful tool but involves consideration of practical limitations and application of appropriate interpretation strategies.
- Normal aging physiology may synergize with the pathophysiology of certain lung diseases to worsen lung function and disease manifestations in geriatric patients.

INTRODUCTION

There are now more Americans older than 65 years than at any other point in US history, and the aging population is expected to increase rapidly over the next decade.[1] Aging influences all aspects of human biology and has characteristic effects on lung structure and function. As with other aspects of human biology, there is heterogeneity of the aging lung with great variability in chronologic, physiologic change among individuals.[2] The main purpose of this article is to review the alterations in lung structure and function that occur with aging in the absence of lung disease. However, insight into these changes in the healthy elderly individual (defined as an individual older than 65 years) can be applied to increase understanding of the manifestations of lung disease in geriatric patients. Whether such knowledge can impact the treatment or treatment response in geriatric lung disease is not currently known.

No disclosures.
Department of Medicine, Division of Pulmonary, Critical Care and Sleep Medicine, Icahn School of Medicine at Mount Sinai, One Gustave L. Levy Place, Box #1232, New York, NY, USA
E-mail address: gwen.skloot@mssm.edu

Clin Geriatr Med 33 (2017) 447–457
http://dx.doi.org/10.1016/j.cger.2017.06.001
0749-0690/17/© 2017 Elsevier Inc. All rights reserved.

geriatric.theclinics.com

STRUCTURAL CHANGES IN LUNG ARCHITECTURE ASSOCIATED WITH AGING

With aging, there are changes in the collagen fiber network that provides support for alveolar structure. These collagen fibers coil around the alveolar ducts and adjacent alveoli and prevent them from collapsing during inflation and deflation of the lung.[3] Alterations in the network of collagen fibers with aging lead to alveolar duct dilation and homogeneous enlargement of alveolar air spaces[3–7] (**Fig. 1**). It is important to distinguish these findings in the senile lung from emphysema. In the latter condition, there is associated inflammation and alveolar wall destruction.[5]

Another important factor that helps to stabilize the alveoli is the production of a substance called surfactant by cells that line the alveoli. Surfactant reduces the surface tension within the alveoli, counteracting their tendency to collapse.[8,9] There is no evidence that the properties of surfactant change with aging.[10] Surface tension is inversely related to alveolar size. Thus, a consequence of alveolar enlargement in the elderly is a reduction in alveolar surface tension leading to a more compliant or distensible lung.

EXTRAPULMONARY STRUCTURAL CHANGES ASSOCIATED WITH AGING

Thoracic shape changes with normal aging with a tendency toward kyphosis due to loss of vertebral body height and even collapse of vertebral bodies.[3,11] There is also increased convexity of the sternum; together, these structural changes result in a greater anteroposterior diameter of the thorax.[3] Chest wall compliance decreases because of the spinal changes, stiffening of the rib cage, and reduced thickness of the parietal (ie, chest wall) muscles.[3,5,7,12,13] In addition, the modifications in the chest wall result in decreased curvature of the diaphragm.[13–15] Finally, there is a loss of respiratory muscle mass. Collectively, these changes place the older individual at a disadvantage in terms of the normal mechanics of breathing. **Box 1** summarizes the structural changes that occur in the respiratory system with aging. These changes are often interrelated with compounded effects.

AGE-RELATED CHANGES IN RESPIRATORY MECHANICS IMPACT EXPIRATORY FLOW AND LUNG VOLUMES

Changes in respiratory mechanics lead to predictable alterations in lung function (**Fig. 2**). A more compliant lung has decreased elastic recoil pressure (ie, the deflation

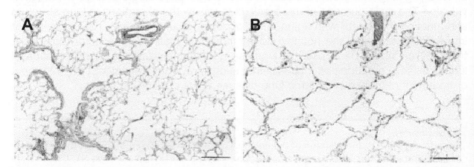

Fig. 1. Lung parenchyma from a 29-year-old nonsmoker (A) compared with that of a 100-year-old nonsmoker (B). Note the presence of alveolar dilation in the elderly subject. (*Adapted from* Janssens JP, Pache JC, Nicod LP. Physiological changes in respiratory function associated with ageing. Eur Respir J 1999;13:197–205; with permission.)

Box 1
Changes in the respiratory system with aging

Changes in lung structure
  Altered collagen fiber network
    ↓
  Dilated alveolar ducts and enlargement of alveoli
    ↓
  Loss of elastic recoil of the lungs

Changes in extrapulmonary structure
  Decreased chest wall compliance
  • Reduced thickness of the parietal muscles
  • Degenerative changes of the spine (eg, kyphosis)
  • Stiffening of the rib cage
  Increased anteroposterior diameter of the chest
  Decreased curvature of the diaphragm
  Decreased respiratory muscle mass

---

force of the lung). The loss of elastic recoil pressure, in turn, will affect expiratory flows and lung volumes.

Healthy nonsmokers lose approximately 30 mL of their forced expiratory volume in 1 second (FEV_1) as assessed by spirometry every year beginning after 30 years of age.[3,4,12] The forced vital capacity (FVC) also decreases with aging. There is an accelerated decline in both FEV_1 and in FVC between 65 and 93 years of age.[16] The FEV_1/FVC ratio characteristically declines with aging producing a flow volume loop in which the expiratory limb seems more obstructed or scooped out (**Fig. 3**).

The changes in respiratory mechanics that lead to decreased airway caliber (and decreased expiratory flows) in the elderly may also explain another observed phenomenon of aging. Young, healthy individuals have the ability to dilate their airways following inhalation of a constrictive substance (ie, such as methacholine). Scichilone and colleagues[17] have demonstrated that this beneficial effect of lung inflation diminishes with aging. Whether this finding relates to the reduced elastic recoil pressure of the lungs in the elderly, to stiffening of the chest wall, or to decreased force generating ability of the respiratory muscles is not known. Diminished elastic recoil of the lungs

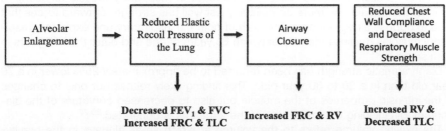

Fig. 2. Changes in respiratory mechanics lead to predictable changes in lung function. The reduction in elastic recoil pressure with aging causes a decrease in forced expiratory volume in 1 second (FEV_1) and forced vital capacity (FVC) as well as an increase in functional residual capacity (FRC) and total lung capacity (TLC). The decreased elastic recoil pressure facilitates airway closure, which increases air trapping (ie, FRC and residual volume [RV] increase). Reduced chest wall compliance and decreased respiratory muscle strength increase RV but tend to decrease TLC so that the net effect on TLC is negligible.

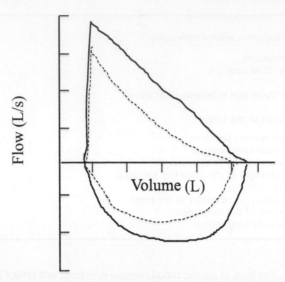

Fig. 3. The expiratory limb of the flow volume loop in an elderly subject (*dashed line*) suggests obstruction to airflow by its convex or scooped-out appearance in contrast to the flow volume loop from a younger subject (*solid line*).

could, in turn, reduce the interdependence between the airway and surrounding lung parenchyma that tends to maintain airway patency. One can speculate that a decrease in the protective function of lung inflation may lead to an increase in bronchial hyperresponsiveness in the aging adult. In fact, in a subsequent study, Scichilone and colleagues[18] found a positive association between aging and airway hyperresponsiveness, although not all the studies evaluated confirmed this association.

Changes in lung volumes also occur with normal aging, as a result of the altered mechanics of breathing. Residual volume (RV), which is the volume of air remaining in the lungs after complete exhalation (ie, often referred to as trapped air), increases by approximately 50% between 20 and 70 years of age.[19] This phenomenon can be explained by premature airway closure. The airways close earlier because of the reduced elastic recoil of the lungs combined with a decrease in chest wall compliance (ie, a stiffer chest wall) and in respiratory muscle strength (ie, related not only to loss of respiratory muscle mass but also to a decrease in respiratory muscle function). In younger individuals, the more compliant chest wall has stronger outward forces that tend to oppose airway closure. Strength of both the inspiratory and expiratory respiratory muscles declines steadily between 65 years of age and older than 85 years in both sexes.[20,21]

Diaphragmatic strength has been reported to be approximately 25% lower in a 76 year old than in a 20 to 30 year old.[3] This finding likely relates not only to changes in the intrinsic properties of the muscle but also to decreased curvature of the diaphragm, diminishing the magnitude of the force that is generated.[20,22]

The closing volume refers to the volume at which small airways in the gravity-dependent areas of the lung begin to close during expiration.[5,21,23] In those aged 65 years or older, the closing volume approaches the seated functional residual capacity (FRC)[5,21]; in other words, the small airways of elderly individuals begin to close even during normal quiet breathing at rest.

The FRC increases with aging as a result of the increase in RV. Total lung capacity (TLC) remains relatively static because the increased RV is opposed by the reduced vital capacity (ie, TLC represents the sum of the RV and vital capacity).[3,6,24] In addition, as seen in **Fig. 2**, although reduced elastic recoil pressure of the lung tends to increase TLC, this is counterbalanced by the decrease in TLC related to reduced chest wall compliance and respiratory muscle strength.[24]

AGE-RELATED CHANGES IN GAS EXCHANGE

The relationship between alveolar ventilation (VA) and pulmonary capillary perfusion (ie, ventilation-perfusion [V/Q] matching) determines the ability of the lung to exchange carbon dioxide and oxygen. The increased closing volume in the elderly with closure of terminal airways even at FRC enhances V/Q mismatch due to ventilation defects.[5,21,23] Such ventilation defects have been visualized using hyperpolarized[3] helium MRI studies.[25] Whereas MRI demonstrates homogeneous lung filling in healthy young individuals, older lifelong nonsmokers have ventilation defects observed in the lung periphery as well as in dependent areas, corresponding to the location of small airway closure.[26] Because maximally effective gas exchange depends on the matching of ventilation with lung perfusion, these low V/Q zones have been hypothesized to be an important mechanism for the age-related decline in Pao_2 and the increase in the alveolar-arterial gradient.[21] Although the existence of low V/Q zones may be one factor in gas exchange abnormalities in the elderly, other studies emphasize the presence of V/Q inequality in general[5,24] with a heterogeneous distribution of lung units having both high and low V/Q ratios. V/Q inequality combined with stiffening of the pulmonary vasculature[27] has been associated with increases in pulmonary artery systolic pressure with aging. In addition, high V/Q zones lead to an increase in dead space ventilation in the elderly (ie, areas of the lung that are ventilated but not perfused).[24] Thus, to maintain the $Paco_2$ in the normal range, older individuals must increase their total minute ventilation (VE) in order to maintain VA, the part of ventilation that contributes to elimination of carbon dioxide.[5] In conjunction with the age-related increase in V/Q inequality, there is a decrease in diffusion capacity of the lung for carbon monoxide (DLCO). DLCO is a measure of the transfer ability of oxygen across the alveolar-capillary membrane; the reduction with aging may relate to decline in alveolar surface area, in the density of lung capillaries, and in the pulmonary capillary blood volume.[5,21,27–30] **Fig. 4** delineates the changes in gas exchange that occur with aging and the factors that may contribute to these changes.

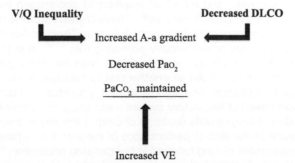

Fig. 4. The changes in gas exchange that occur with aging relate to V/Q inequality and decreases in DLCO. The alveolar-arterial oxygen gradient (A-a gradient) increases in the elderly, whereas Pao_2 decreases. $Paco_2$ is maintained because of increased VE to compensate for increases in the dead space fraction and possible decreased neural sensitivity to an elevated $Paco_2$.

ALTERATIONS IN EXERCISE PHYSIOLOGY RELATED TO AGING

Given the alterations in resting lung function that occur with aging, it is not surprising to find changes in exercise physiology in the older adult. Older individuals experience an increase in expiratory flow limitation during exercise with an increase in end expiratory lung volume.[27] This finding, combined with an elevated dead space fraction (ie, the ratio of dead space to tidal volume) at rest, increases the work of breathing in the elderly.[21,27,31] The normal response to exercise involves an early increase in tidal volume with subsequent increase in respiratory rate when the tidal volume reaches a plateau. The respiratory pattern in the elderly is characterized by higher respiratory rates and lower tidal volumes[21] perhaps, in part, because of the increased stiffness of the chest wall. The abdominal muscles also play a greater role during exercise in older adults than in younger individuals.

There is some controversy in terms of the ventilatory responses to carbon dioxide and oxygen in the elderly at rest. Some studies indicate that older individuals have a blunted response to hypercapnia and hypoxia, suggesting an attenuated ability to integrate signals received from chemoreceptors and mechanoreceptors and to respond with appropriate neural activity; but others do not demonstrate these findings.[21] During exercise, there is evidence that the elderly may be more responsive to carbon dioxide production than younger individuals.[21,32,33] This response is likely linked to the increased dead space to tidal volume ratio. Thus, per unit of carbon dioxide produced, total VE is higher during exercise in the elderly.[32] Maximal oxygen consumption, a global measure of exercise capacity, decreases with advancing age; but this is predominantly a result of cardiovascular factors and, to some extent, loss of muscle mass.[21,31,34] More recent evidence suggests that ventilatory factors may also play a role.[31] It is noteworthy that fit elderly individuals can achieve levels of maximal oxygen consumption that exceed those of middle-aged untrained men.[35] Thus, pulmonary rehabilitation programs can play an important role in increasing exercise capacity in elderly individuals.[21,36]

LUNG FUNCTION TESTING IN THE ELDERLY

Routine lung function testing in the elderly is generally useful to assess pulmonary physiology, but there are several caveats to consider. It may be difficult for some geriatric patients to perform pulmonary function tests that involve forceful breathing maneuvers with complete exhalation to residual volume. Elderly patients can require 10 to 20 seconds to fully exhale, and the effort required to accomplish this may lead to exhaustion and even to syncope.[37] Studies[38,39] have shown that 80% or more of older individuals can perform spirometry that meets American Thoracic Society's standards but frail older patients may have difficulty achieving this.[40–42] In such cases, surrogates of the FEV_1/FVC, such as the FEV_1/FEV_6, may be more easily obtainable because less effort is required. An alternative test to consider is impulse oscillation testing (or forced oscillation testing). This test provides a completely effort-independent assessment of respiratory system mechanics and offers insight into abnormalities in different lung regions (ie, large or central airways vs small or peripheral airways).[43] Because of the ease of performance of the test, it may have utility, particularly in the measurement of lung function in the geriatric population.[44]

Because some elderly individuals may have difficulty performing respiratory tests that involve forced expiration, bronchoprovocation protocols to assess for airway hyperresponsiveness (ie, asthma) may be challenging. These tests typically require multiple sets of repeated spirometry maneuvers.[19] During interpretation of bronchoprovocation testing in the elderly, attention should be paid to the quality of the spirometry efforts given the potential for fatigue.[45] Also, it should be noted that lower lung function in the elderly may, in some circumstances, preclude performance of such tests. In general, however, measurement of bronchial responsiveness is feasible and of clinical value in older patients.

A second caveat in terms of geriatric lung function testing relates to the interpretation of the tests rather than to the breathing maneuvers themselves. Age-adjusted values are essential to the analysis of results. Before the publication of reference standards for spirometry from the Global Lung Function Initiative,[46] interpretation of spirometry in individuals older than 80 years was imperfect. Overdiagnosis of respiratory impairment based on the FEV_1/FVC was a particular problem. The Global Lung Function Initiative extended the age incorporated into spirometry reference sets to 95 years. Although this represents an advance in the assessment of spirometry in the elderly, data for nonwhite individuals and for those older than 75 years are limited.[19] This author is not aware of any comparable reference equations applicable to lung volume or DLCO testing.

SYNERGISTIC EFFECT OF AGE-RELATED CHANGES IN LUNG STRUCTURE AND FUNCTION ON LUNG DISEASE

The pulmonary physiologic changes of the aging lung may synergize with the pathologic changes of various lung diseases to affect lung structure and function. Such synergistic effects may lead to more severe manifestations of lung disease in the elderly. Loss of elastic recoil of the lung is a prominent feature of aging and is also a characteristic feature of chronic asthma[47,48] and chronic obstructive pulmonary disease[49] regardless of aging. This may explain the accelerated decline in FEV_1 in asthma that has been noted longitudinally in some population studies.[50,51] The presence of alveolar enlargement in the aged adult likely coexists with destruction of alveolar walls and the inflammatory infiltrate found in patients with emphysema.

Aging leads to changes in the expression of transforming growth factor-β and extracellular matrix composition. These changes may partially explain the increased incidence of fibrotic lung disorders in the elderly.[52] Although aging typically decreases the elastic recoil of the lung, this phenomenon is likely overshadowed by the opposing effect of fibrotic lung disease. In fibrotic lung disease, elastic recoil pressure is increased[53] because of the overall stiffening of the parenchyma. Thus, expiratory flows are typically increased relative to volume. Although TLC is characteristically maintained with normal aging, because the increased RV is counterbalanced by the decrease in vital capacity, this is not the case in the older individual with fibrotic lung disease given the exaggerated decrease in vital capacity in such a setting. Interestingly, in patients with combined emphysema and interstitial lung disease,[54] lung volumes and expiratory flows have been found to be normal presumably because the effect of each condition on elastic recoil pressure is profound.

Aging is associated with changes in the pulmonary circulation that occur in response to increased dead space ventilation and V/Q mismatch as well as to general stiffening of the pulmonary vasculature.[5,27] One such consequence is an increase in pulmonary arterial systolic pressure.[55] Although the increase in pulmonary pressures with aging is not dramatic, the degree of pulmonary hypertension may be accentuated in the elderly adult with severe underlying lung disease (eg, emphysema, interstitial lung disease, and so forth).[56] This accentuation may be particularly pertinent during exercise because pulmonary hypertension with exercise is not uncommonly seen in otherwise healthy geriatric patients.[55] The effects on the pulmonary circulation due to aging combined with severe lung disease may worsen gas exchange and increase the work of breathing.

The combination of aging and the obese state has important effects on respiratory anatomy and physiology.[57] Obesity is fairly common in the elderly, affecting more than one-third of adults older than 65 years.[31,58] Obesity, independent of lung disease, is characterized by peripheral airways dysfunction as measured by forced oscillation testing.[59] The author's group has demonstrated the presence of increased small airways resistance in obesity as well as increased low frequency reactance area, another forced oscillation measure that reflects peripheral lung stiffness. Thus, peripheral airway dysfunction is common to both obesity and aging and, in combination, may enhance the tendency toward reduced airway caliber.

LUNG STRUCTURAL CHANGES IN THE ELDERLY AND INHALED THERAPY

In a study on modeling particle deposition as a function of age,[60] changes in tissue elasticity were thought to be important, although the investigators noted that the effect of adult aging-related phenomena on inhaled aerosol deposition has not been delineated and certainly not quantified. One might speculate that the closure of small airways in the elderly even at FRC might prevent inhaled therapy from reaching the target area in older individuals with obstructive lung disease. It is possible that such individuals may not respond as well to existing therapies and that different formulations with the anatomic changes in mind might be more effective.

SUMMARY

Characteristic changes occur in lung structure and function in the setting of the normal aging process. Alterations in respiratory mechanics combined with changes in the pulmonary circulation lead to a reduction in expiratory flows, an increase in closing volume, and decreases in gas exchange. These findings impact lung function both at rest and during exercise. When assessing lung function in the aged adult, there are several issues to consider, including (1) choosing the most appropriate type of test (ie, considering patients' ability to perform traditional forced breathing maneuvers), (2) interpreting the test using validated age-adjusted values when available (ie, for spirometry), and (3) accepting the fact that interpretation of certain lung function tests may be limited by the absence of age-appropriate values (ie, for lung volume testing and DLCO). Geriatric patients are likely more vulnerable to the effects of lung disease given the unfavorable physiologic modifications that occur even in the healthy individual. Effects due to aging may not always be distinguishable from those due to a specific lung disease, particularly when these effects are synergistic. It is important to recognize that the normal aging process may impact the manifestations of lung disease and potentially even the response to treatment.

REFERENCES

1. Vincent GK, Velkoff VA, Bureau USC. The next four decades: the older population in the United States: 2010 to 2050. Washington, DC: U.S. Dept. of Commerce, Economics and Statistics Administration, U.S. Census Bureau; 2010.
2. Hanania NA, King MJ, Braman SS, et al. Asthma in the elderly: current understanding and future research needs–a report of a National Institute on Aging (NIA) workshop. J Allergy Clin Immunol 2011;128:S4–24.
3. Miller MR. Structural and physiological age-associated changes in aging lungs. Semin Respir Crit Care Med 2010;31:521–7.

4. Yanez A, Cho SH, Soriano JB, et al. Asthma in the elderly: what we know and what we have yet to know. World Allergy Organ J 2014;7:8.

5. Vaz Fragoso CA, Gill TM. Respiratory impairment and the aging lung: a novel paradigm for assessing pulmonary function. J Gerontol A Biol Sci Med Sci 2012;67:264–75.

6. Janssens JP, Pache JC, Nicod LP. Physiological changes in respiratory function associated with ageing. Eur Respir J 1999;13:197–205.

7. Hochhegger B, Meirelles GS, Irion K, et al. The chest and aging: radiological findings. J Bras Pneumol 2012;38:656–65.

8. Possmayer F, Hall SB, Haller T, et al. Recent advances in alveolar biology: some new looks at the alveolar interface. Respir Physiol Neurobiol 2010;173(Suppl):S55–64.

9. Griese M. Pulmonary surfactant in health and human lung diseases: state of the art. Eur Respir J 1999;13:1455–76.

10. Rebello CM, Jobe AH, Eisele JW, et al. Alveolar and tissue surfactant pool sizes in humans. Am J Respir Crit Care Med 1996;154:625–8.

11. Kado DM, Prenovost K, Crandall C. Narrative review: hyperkyphosis in older persons. Ann Intern Med 2007;147:330–8.

12. Sharma G, Goodwin J. Effect of aging on respiratory system physiology and immunology. Clin Interv Aging 2006;1:253–60.

13. Lowery EM, Brubaker AL, Kuhlmann E, et al. The aging lung. Clin Interv Aging 2013;8:1489–96.

14. Zaugg M, Lucchinetti E. Respiratory function in the elderly. Anesthesiol Clin North America 2000;18:47–58, vi.

15. Sprung J, Gajic O, Warner DO. Review article: age related alterations in respiratory function - anesthetic considerations. Can J Anaesth 2006;53:1244–57.

16. Sorino C, Battaglia S, Scichilone N, et al. Diagnosis of airway obstruction in the elderly: contribution of the SARA study. Int J Chron Obstruct Pulmon Dis 2012;7:389–95.

17. Scichilone N, Marchese R, Catalano F, et al. The bronchodilatory effect of deep inspiration diminishes with aging. Respir Med 2004;98:838–43.

18. Scichilone N, Messina M, Battaglia S, et al. Airway hyperresponsiveness in the elderly: prevalence and clinical implications. Eur Respir J 2005;25:364–75.

19. Skloot GS, Busse PJ, Braman SS, et al. An official American Thoracic Society workshop report: evaluation and management of asthma in the elderly. Ann Am Thorac Soc 2016;13:2064–77.

20. Kelley RC, Ferreira LF. Diaphragm abnormalities in heart failure and aging: mechanisms and integration of cardiovascular and respiratory pathophysiology. Heart Fail Rev 2016;22(2):191–207.

21. Janssens JP. Aging of the respiratory system: impact on pulmonary function tests and adaptation to exertion. Clin Chest Med 2005;26:469–84, vi-vii.

22. Gosselin LE, Johnson BD, Sieck GC. Age-related changes in diaphragm muscle contractile properties and myosin heavy chain isoforms. Am J Respir Crit Care Med 1994;150:174–8.

23. Leblanc P, Ruff F, Milic-Emili J. Effects of age and body position on "airway closure" in man. J Appl Physiol 1970;28:448–51.

24. Lalley PM. The aging respiratory system–pulmonary structure, function and neural control. Respir Physiol Neurobiol 2013;187:199–210.

25. Sheikh K, Paulin GA, Svenningsen S, et al. Pulmonary ventilation defects in older never-smokers. J Appl Physiol (1985) 2014;117:297–306.

26. Parraga G, Mathew L, Etemad-Rezai R, et al. Hyperpolarized 3He magnetic resonance imaging of ventilation defects in healthy elderly volunteers: initial findings at 3.0 Tesla. Acad Radiol 2008;15:776–85.

27. Taylor BJ, Johnson BD. The pulmonary circulation and exercise responses in the elderly. Semin Respir Crit Care Med 2010;31:528–38.

28. Georges R, Saumon G, Loiseau A. The relationship of age to pulmonary membrane conductance and capillary blood volume. Am Rev Respir Dis 1978;117: 1069–78.

29. Chang SC, Chang HI, Liu SY, et al. Effects of body position and age on membrane diffusing capacity and pulmonary capillary blood volume. Chest 1992; 102:139–42.

30. Butler C 2nd, Kleinerman J. Capillary density: alveolar diameter, a morphometric approach to ventilation and perfusion. Am Rev Respir Dis 1970;102:886–94.

31. Roman MA, Rossiter HB, Casaburi R. Exercise, ageing and the lung. Eur Respir J 2016;48:1471–86.

32. Poulin MJ, Cunningham DA, Paterson DH, et al. Ventilatory response to exercise in men and women 55 to 86 years of age. Am J Respir Crit Care Med 1994;149: 408–15.

33. Inbar O, Oren A, Scheinowitz M, et al. Normal cardiopulmonary responses during incremental exercise in 20- to 70-yr-old men. Med Sci Sports Exerc 1994;26: 538–46.

34. Stamford BA. Exercise and the elderly. Exerc Sport Sci Rev 1988;16:341–79.

35. Heath GW, Hagberg JM, Ehsani AA, et al. A physiological comparison of young and older endurance athletes. J Appl Physiol Respir Environ Exerc Physiol 1981; 51:634–40.

36. Bichay AA, Ramirez JM, Nunez VM, et al. Efficacy of treadmill exercises on arterial blood oxygenation, oxygen consumption and walking distance in healthy elderly people: a controlled trial. BMC Geriatr 2016;16:110.

37. Melbye H, Medbo A, Crockett A. The FEV1/FEV6 ratio is a good substitute for the FEV1/FVC ratio in the elderly. Prim Care Respir J 2006;15:294–8.

38. Luoto JA, Elmstahl S, Wollmer P, et al. Incidence of airflow limitation in subjects 65-100 years of age. Eur Respir J 2016;47:461–72.

39. Bellia V, Battaglia S, Matera MG, et al. The use of bronchodilators in the treatment of airway obstruction in elderly patients. Pulm Pharmacol Ther 2006;19:311–9.

40. Bellia V, Pistelli R, Catalano F, et al. Quality control of spirometry in the elderly. The SA.R.A. study. SAlute respiration nell'Anziano = respiratory health in the elderly. Am J Respir Crit Care Med 2000;161:1094–100.

41. Allen SC, Yeung P. Inability to draw intersecting pentagons as a predictor of unsatisfactory spirometry technique in elderly hospital inpatients. Age Ageing 2006; 35:304–6.

42. Allen SC, Ragab S. Ability to learn inhaler technique in relation to cognitive scores and tests of praxis in old age. Postgrad Med J 2002;78:37–9.

43. Desiraju K, Agrawal A. Impulse oscillometry: the state-of-art for lung function testing. Lung India 2016;33:410–6.

44. Chalker RB, Celli BR. Special considerations in the elderly patient. Clin Chest Med 1993;14:437–52.

45. Connolly MJ, Crowley JJ, Charan NB, et al. Reduced subjective awareness of bronchoconstriction provoked by methacholine in elderly asthmatic and normal subjects as measured on a simple awareness scale. Thorax 1992;47:410–3.

46. Quanjer PH, Stanojevic S, Cole TJ, et al. Multi-ethnic reference values for spirometry for the 3-95-yr age range: the global lung function 2012 equations. Eur Respir J 2012;40:1324–43.
47. Gelb AF, Yamamoto A, Verbeken EK, et al. Unraveling the pathophysiology of the asthma-COPD overlap syndrome: unsuspected mild centrilobular emphysema is responsible for loss of lung elastic recoil in never smokers with asthma with persistent expiratory airflow limitation. Chest 2015;148:313–20.
48. Gelb AF, Licuanan J, Shinar CM, et al. Unsuspected loss of lung elastic recoil in chronic persistent asthma. Chest 2002;121:715–21.
49. Di Petta A. Pathogenesis of pulmonary emphysema - cellular and molecular events. Einstein (Sao Paulo) 2010;8:248–51.
50. James AL, Palmer LJ, Kicic E, et al. Decline in lung function in the Busselton Health Study: the effects of asthma and cigarette smoking. Am J Respir Crit Care Med 2005;171:109–14.
51. Bai TR, Cooper J, Koelmeyer T, et al. The effect of age and duration of disease on airway structure in fatal asthma. Am J Respir Crit Care Med 2000;162:663–9.
52. Selman M, Rojas M, Mora AL, et al. Aging and interstitial lung diseases: unraveling an old forgotten player in the pathogenesis of lung fibrosis. Semin Respir Crit Care Med 2010;31:607–17.
53. Hanley ME, King TE Jr, Schwarz MI, et al. The impact of smoking on mechanical properties of the lungs in idiopathic pulmonary fibrosis and sarcoidosis. Am Rev Respir Dis 1991;144:1102–6.
54. Heathcote KL, Cockcroft DW, Fladeland DA, et al. Normal expiratory flow rate and lung volumes in patients with combined emphysema and interstitial lung disease: a case series and literature review. Can Respir J 2011;18:e73–6.
55. Berra G, Noble S, Soccal PM, et al. Pulmonary hypertension in the elderly: a different disease? Breathe (Sheff) 2016;12:43–9.
56. Brewis MJ, Church AC, Johnson MK, et al. Severe pulmonary hypertension in lung disease: phenotypes and response to treatment. Eur Respir J 2015;46:1378–89.
57. Harrington J, Lee-Chiong T. Obesity and aging. Clin Chest Med 2009;30:609–14, x.
58. Fakhouri TH, Ogden CL, Carroll MD, et al. Prevalence of obesity among older adults in the United States, 2007-2010. NCHS Data Brief 2012;1–8.
59. Skloot G, Schechter C, Desai A, et al. Impaired response to deep inspiration in obesity. J Appl Physiol (1985) 2011;111:726–34.
60. Phalen RF, Oldham MJ. Methods for modeling particle deposition as a function of age. Respir Physiol 2001;128:119–30.

Inflammaging and the Lung

Elizabeth J. Kovacs, PhD[a],*, Devin M. Boe, BA[b], Lisbeth A. Boule, PhD[c],
Brenda J. Curtis, PhD[d]

KEYWORDS

- Inflammaging • Elderly • Infection • Host defense • Macrophage • Neutrophils
- Inflammation • Immunosenescence

KEY POINTS

- Age-dependent changes in immune responses cause increased morbidity and mortality in the elderly.
- Inflammaging causes immunosenescence.
- Intestinal permeability in the elderly may be responsible for inflammaging.
- The ability of alveolar macrophages to maintain pulmonary homeostasis following clearance of infection is reduced in the aged.

INTRODUCTION

With advanced age, there are changes in multiple biologic systems[1] including the immune system. Alterations in innate and adaptive immune cells in the aged have been noted.[2,3] In brief, the age-dependent effects on the innate immune response include diminished pathogen recognition, chemotaxis, and phagocytosis, and in adaptive

Disclosure: This work was funded in part by grants from the National Institutes of Health (R01 AG018859; R01 GM115257 and T32 AG000279).
[a] Division of GI, Trauma and Endocrine Surgery, Department of Surgery, Mucosal Inflammation Program, GILIIP (GI, Liver and Innate Immunity Program), Graduate Program in Immunology, IMAGE (Investigations in Metabolism, Aging, Gender and Exercise), University of Colorado Denver, Anschutz Medical Campus, 12700 East 19th Avenue, Research Complex 2, Mailstop #8620, Aurora, CO 80045, USA; [b] Division of GI, Trauma and Endocrine Surgery, Department of Surgery, Mucosal Inflammation Program, Graduate Program in Immunology, University of Colorado Denver, Anschutz Medical Campus, 12700 East 19th Avenue, Research Complex 2, Room 6460, Aurora, CO 80045, USA; [c] Division of GI, Trauma and Endocrine Surgery, Department of Surgery, Mucosal Inflammation Program, IMAGE, University of Colorado Denver, Anschutz Medical Campus, 12700 East 19th Avenue, Research Complex 2, Room 6460, Aurora, CO 80045, USA; [d] Division of GI, Trauma and Endocrine Surgery, Department of Surgery, Mucosal Inflammation Program, IMAGE, University of Colorado Denver, Anschutz Medical Campus, 12700 East 19th Avenue, Research Complex 2, Room 6018, Aurora, CO 80045, USA
* Corresponding author.
E-mail address: elizabeth.kovacs@ucdenver.edu

immunity, declining numbers of naive T lymphocytes and reduced cytotoxicity and antibody quality and quantity.[2] Vaccine efficacy is reduced in the elderly, as are increases in autoimmunity and cancer.[2] Overall, these immune defects, referred to collectively as immunosenescence, render the host less able to withstand injury or infection relative to younger individuals.

Among the hallmarks of the aging immune system is the persistent low-grade proinflammatory state characterized by heightened basal levels of proinflammatory mediators in the blood.[4] Because of this association of advanced age and inflammation, Claudio Franceschi coined the term "inflammaging" in 2000.[4] Franceschi and coworkers[4] have reported that, even in healthy aged subjects without confirmed ailments, there is an elevated basal level of proinflammatory mediators, including interleukin (IL)-1β, IL-6, and tumor necrosis factor-α. The elevated levels of these and other proinflammatory factors in the aged can have local and systemic consequences, none of which are ultimately beneficial to the host. This rise in circulating levels of proinflammatory cytokines and other factors is thought by some to be a driving factor in the development and maintenance of immunosenescence[4,5] and contribute to chronic diseases of the lung and other organs.[6–8] In this review, the focus is on inflammaging, immunosenescence, and the lung, but it should be noted that many of the age-dependent changes are neither limited to nor likely to be caused by changes in the aging lung itself, and most of these changes are not observed unless the host is challenged by some form of stressor, such as an injury or infection.

CHANGES IN THE LUNG WITH ADVANCED AGE

A wide range of pulmonary parameters that influence lung immunity are altered with advanced age as described in **Table 1**.

INNATE IMMUNE CELLS OF THE LUNG AND CHANGES WITH ADVANCED AGE
Macrophages

The primary resident innate immune cell in the airway is the alveolar macrophage. This multifaceted cell serves as the first line of defense against invading pathogens and

Table 1
Aging of the lung

Lung Functions That Are Changed with Age	Reference
↓ Mucociliary escalator: reduced ability to clear microbes and debris from the airway	9,10
↑ Expression of proteins associated with bacteria attachment and infiltration in the pulmonary epithelial cells, including polymeric immunoglobulin receptor and platelet-activating factor receptor	11,12
↑ Expression of markers of cellular senescence	6,13
↓ Epithelial expression of antimicrobial peptides	14,15
↑ Levels of complement and surfactant proteins	15
↑ Proteostasis (and the loss of ability of cells from the aged to properly control protein abundance, proper folding, and degradation)	16,17
↑ Susceptibility to pulmonary infections	2,11,12,18–22
Dysbiosis (or the imbalance) of the pulmonary microbiome in the absence of infection and after infection	23–28

plays a critical role in lung immunologic homeostasis. Macrophages are capable of initiating and resolving an inflammatory response.[29–31] This ability to play divergent roles is caused by macrophage plasticity. Macrophages can adapt and even change phenotype in response to environmental cues, enabling them to adapt to varying conditions and perform a plethora of diverse functions.[32–35] Historically, this stimulus-induced shift in macrophage phenotype was referred to as M1 and M2 phenotypes with M1 being proinflammatory and M2 anti-inflammatory.[36,37] However, because of poor definition and inconsistencies in the cell surface markers defining these two phenotypes, a group of expert macrophage research investigators recently redefined macrophage classification terminology so that they are more narrowly classified based on the source of the macrophages and activation stimuli, and the specific group of markers associated with the particular activation phenotype.[38] Regardless of nomenclature, under resting conditions, alveolar macrophages maintain an anti-inflammatory profile to keep the pulmonary airway in check and are capable of rapidly springing into action, becoming strongly proinflammatory when alerted by the presence of foreign material (**Fig. 1**). After pathogen clearance, the ability of alveolar macrophages to promote resolution and return to an anti-inflammatory resting phenotype is equally important for maintenance of lung homeostasis.

Multiple factors are involved in the resolution of inflammation in the lung. These include but are not limited to (1) clearance of the pathogen or debris; (2) reduced production of neutrophil chemokines; and (3) removal of apoptotic cells, including effete neutrophils. All of these processes are orchestrated by alveolar macrophages.[39] It should be noted that the inability of macrophages to perform these functions can result in prolonged inflammation, which if left unchecked can result in damage to

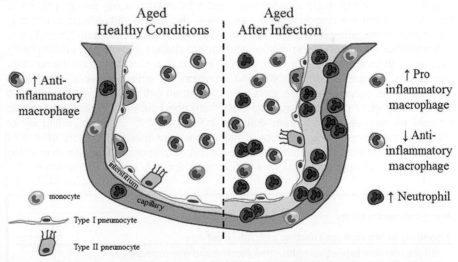

Fig. 1. Innate immune phenotype of the aged lung. Regardless of age, under healthy conditions, the major leukocyte of the distal lung is the alveolar macrophage. These multifaceted cells exist in an anti-inflammatory state to limit inflammation and maintain pulmonary homeostasis. A variety of pathogenic conditions alter alveolar macrophage function. In the young, alveolar macrophages can rapidly respond to external stimuli, such as bacteria; clear infections; and return to their anti-inflammatory state. In contrast, in the elderly, alveolar macrophages fail to mount an adequate response to infectious insult, are slow at recruiting neutrophils to help combat the respiratory pathogens, and are unable to return to their anti-inflammatory phenotype, thus leaving the lung in a compromised state.

lung tissue.[40] Central to the restoration of pulmonary homeostasis is the removal of neutrophils, which is associated with a shift in alveolar macrophages phenotype to an anti-inflammatory profile.[39]

With advanced age, it is clear that the ability of macrophages to perform their normal functions is impaired and that inflammaging plays a role in this altered response despite the lack of change in macrophage number. A comprehensive review of macrophage function and aging is available.[36] In brief, in vivo and in vitro studies conducted in humans and in various animal models suggest that many but not all of the functions of macrophages are slowed or diminished in magnitude in the aged, leaving the host unable to shift between phenotypes when needed.[2,33,36] Some of the better documented age-dependent changes in macrophage function are highlighted in **Table 2**.

Neutrophils

The neutrophil is a key innate immune cell that is often the first cell type to be recruited to sites of injury and infection. Neutrophils are capable of performing a variety of antimicrobial functions that play a critical role in removing pathogens from tissues during the early stages of lung infections. Within minutes after recognition of foreign material, macrophages become activated and initiate a cascade of events that includes the release of chemoattractant cytokines that recruit neutrophils. Working together, macrophages and neutrophils join forces to remove and destroy infectious organisms.[58,59] Neutrophil functions that are altered with advanced age are shown in **Table 3**.

A PARADOX: AGING CAUSES HIGHER CYTOKINE LEVELS IN VIVO, YET REDUCED PRODUCTION BY INFLAMMATORY CELLS IN VITRO

The cellular sources of the mediators responsible for inflammaging remain unknown. Interestingly, there is a disconnect between the in vivo and in vitro effects of stimulation on the inflammatory response in young adult and older subjects and in cells isolated from those subjects. From human and rodent studies in which an inflammatory stimulus, such as lipopolysaccharide, is given in vivo, it is clear that the inflammatory response is of greater magnitude and duration in older subjects relative to younger.[88–90] In contrast, in vitro stimulation of certain cell subsets, including blood monocytes, lung, or peritoneal macrophages from aged subjects, yields lower levels of cytokines relative to cells from younger individuals,[44–46,91,92] suggesting either that monocyte/macrophages are not a major source of these mediators in vivo or that there are additional factors responsible for this discrepancy. The effects of aging on monocyte/macrophage functions were comprehensively reviewed elsewhere.[36]

Table 2 Aging and macrophages	
Alterations in Macrophage Function with Advanced Age	**Reference**
↓ Toll-like receptor expression (mRNA and protein) and downstream signaling (in most but not all studies)	23,41–46
↓ Production of proinflammatory and immunomodulatory cytokines, including tumor necrosis factor-α, IL-6, IL-1β, and CCL2 (monocyte chemoattractant protein-1) after stimulation by various agonists	44–50
↓ Telomere length	51
↑ Regulators of immune signaling, such as A20, a deubiquitinase that, in turn, inhibits toll-like receptor signaling and nuclear factor-κB activation	11,12
↓ Phagocytosis and pathogen clearance	7,49,52–57

Table 3
Aging and neutrophils

Alterations in Neutrophil Function with Advanced Age	Reference
↓ Chemotaxis	60–67
No change in chemokinesis	60
↓ Phagocytosis	62,64,68–75
↓ Production of reactive oxygen species	61,62,64,70,71,76–78
↓ Generation of neutrophil extracellular traps	79–81
↓ Production of proinflammatory cytokines and mediators, including IL-6, IL-8, myeloperoxidase, elastase, and ↑ production of anti-inflammatory cytokines, IL-10	76,82,83
No increase in lifespan following stimulation	83–87

WHAT CAUSES INFLAMMAGING?

There are multiple theories about the origin and perpetuation of inflammaging. Ones that have gained press over time include classical ideas about increased oxidative stress, DNA damage, and telomere shortening.[1,2] In brief, it is believed that with advanced age there is an increase in posttranslational modification of macromolecules including DNA, proteins, and lipids that stimulate leukocytes and other cells to secrete proinflammatory cytokines; and senescence of immune and nonimmune cells leading to an increased release of inflammatory mediators via a senescence-associated secretory phenotype.[1,2] Additionally, a complementary and newer theory about the initiation of inflammaging is emerging and gaining support in the literature. This theory revolves around changes in intestinal permeability that allows bacteria and bacterial products (eg, endotoxin and peptidoglycan) to translocate into the lymphatic system and ultimately the bloodstream where they can trigger the low systemic inflammation in the elderly.

In brief, changes in aged intestine include dysbiosis of intestinal microbiota in animal models of aging and in elderly humans,[93–96] and decreased integrity of the intestinal epithelial cell barrier in mice and humans.[97–102]

AGING, DYSBIOSIS OF INTESTINAL MICROBIOME, AND THE GUT-LIVER-LUNG AXIS

Extensive clinical and experimental evidence reveals that the intestinal barrier integrity plays a role in inflammaging that in turn alters pulmonary inflammation. The gut hypothesis states that heightened intestinal permeability, along with changes in immune function of the gut, results in increased translocation of bacteria and bacterial products.[103–105]

Like the lung, the intestine is an organ that is exposed to the outside environment with a large surface area. Although the lung and intestine provide different biologic functions, they share in common the feature of needing to maintain compartmental barriers that must remain intact to permit normal organ function to occur and to protect the host from invading pathogens. Those barriers are created by the epithelium lining the lumen of the respiratory and gastrointestinal tract. The integrity of tight junctions between adjacent epithelial cells is an essential part of these barriers. In young and the aged, this barrier is maintained in part by the complex interactions between the multiple proteins making up tight junctions, including occludins and claudins, along with multiple adaptor and scaffolding proteins. Under normal conditions, the epithelium maintains a semipermeable barrier permitting passage of smaller molecules while preventing the movement of other materials to its underlying mucosal tissue. Regardless of the organ, breach of the epithelial barrier allows inappropriate access of microbial organisms and debris to the underlying mucosa, which can cause inflammation and tissue damage.[106–109] The integrity of this barrier is perturbed in a plethora of disease states, such as reflux esophagitis, cancer, and inflammatory bowel disease (discussed elsewhere).[108,109]

One mechanism of altering the epithelial status quo is mediated by the enzyme myosin light chain kinase (MLCK), the long 210-kDa form that remains inactive in the cytoplasm of epithelial (and endothelial) cells. When activated, MLCK phosphorylates myosin regulatory light-chain (MLC) at serine 19, allowing it to interact with actin. The interaction between actin and MLC causes cytoskeletal sliding, which disrupts tight junctions and creates a gap in the epithelial barrier,[110,111] thus permitting the uncontrolled flow of fluid, bacteria, bacterial products, and other materials across the epithelial lining.[112,113] Of interest to research on the elderly, the same set of proinflammatory mediators that are elevated in the circulation of the aged and serve as hallmarks of inflammaging, namely IL-1β, IL-6, and tumor necrosis factor-α, can trigger the activation of MLCK. Additionally, in the lung, when MLCK is activated in the capillary lining endothelial cells, it results in paracellular permeability, which can lead to pulmonary edema.[110] One of the consequences of the leakiness of the intestinal epithelium is the translocation of bacteria from the intestinal lumen to the underlying mucosal tissue and to regional lymph nodes. Subsequently, these products can traffic to the liver where they can stimulate production of proinflammatory cytokines (**Fig. 2**). If not appropriately contained by the aging immune system, the dissemination of

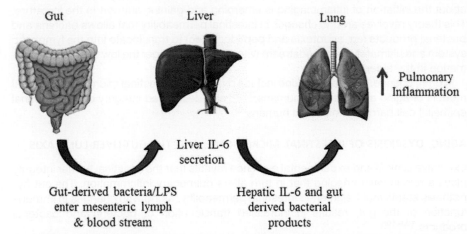

Gut   Liver   Lung

↑ Pulmonary Inflammation

Liver IL-6 secretion

Gut-derived bacteria/LPS enter mesenteric lymph & blood stream

Hepatic IL-6 and gut derived bacterial products

Fig. 2. The gut-liver-lung axis. Under healthy conditions, the epithelial cells lining the intestine maintain tight junctions preventing luminal contents from invading the underlying mucosal tissues. In the aged, it is thought that epithelial cell tight junctions loosen, possibly in response to the presence of the proinflammatory cytokines associated with inflammaging. This loosening of junctional complexes and subsequent increase in paracellular permeability allows gut-derived bacteria, bacterial products, and endotoxins to enter the mesenteric lymph and the bloodstream. Bacteria and their products then trigger Kupffer cells and other cells in the liver to produce and secrete proinflammatory cytokines, including IL-6. Hepatic-derived IL-6, along with the gut-derived bacteria products in the circulation, promotes baseline lung inflammation, which can then be further exacerbated in the aged after injury or infection. LPS, lipopolysaccharide.

bacteria and/or release of bacteria and bacterial products, such as endotoxins, throughout the body can occur, leading to prolonged and exacerbated inflammation in all organs, which likely contributes to increased morbidity and mortality in the aged. Hence, the intestine and its microbial contents can play a critical role in inducing or exacerbating complications in various patient populations[111,114] and in the aged.[101,102,115-117]

SUMMARY AND FUTURE DIRECTIONS

Factors or treatments that reduce inflammaging are of interest to basic and clinical researchers because they may be able to dampen the prolonged and heightened inflammation seen in the elderly after attempting to combat an infection. Thoughts about the design of therapeutic interventions to reduce inflammaging can be directed either at cells themselves or the proinflammatory environment in which they reside. Animal studies involving adoptive transfer of subsets of leukocytes are in progress, as are numerous clinical and basic research studies investigating antioxidant and anti-inflammatory agents to attenuate the overexuberant inflammatory response in the aged. Some believe that taking the indirect approach of reducing intestinal inflammation or restoring the intestinal microbiota may have benefit, but this is not without controversy.[118-120] It would be of interest to determine if patients receiving anti-inflammatory therapies for other conditions have restored intestinal barrier function and if this, in turn, improves systemic responses to the injury or infection in the aged population. Further exploration of these direct and indirect avenues of therapeutic manipulation may be of benefit to the overall health of the aged and with that will likely improve overall lung health of the elderly.

REFERENCES

1. Lopez-Otin C, Blasco MA, Partridge L, et al. The hallmarks of aging. Cell 2013; 153(6):1194–217.
2. Frasca D, Blomberg BB. Inflammaging decreases adaptive and innate immune responses in mice and humans. Biogerontology 2016;17(1):7–19.
3. Shaw AC, Goldstein DR, Montgomery RR. Age-dependent dysregulation of innate immunity. Nat Rev Immunol 2013;13(12):875–87.
4. Franceschi C, Bonafe M, Valensin S, et al. Inflamm-aging. An evolutionary perspective on immunosenescence. Ann N Y Acad Sci 2000;908:244–54.
5. Solana R, Tarazona R, Gayoso I, et al. Innate immunosenescence: effect of aging on cells and receptors of the innate immune system in humans. Semin Immunol 2012;24(5):331–41.
6. Franceschi C, Campisi J. Chronic inflammation (inflammaging) and its potential contribution to age-associated diseases. J Gerontol A Biol Sci Med Sci 2014; 69(Suppl 1):S4–9.
7. Hearps AC, Martin GE, Angelovich TA, et al. Aging is associated with chronic innate immune activation and dysregulation of monocyte phenotype and function. Aging Cell 2012;11(5):867–75.
8. Murray MA, Chotirmall SH. The impact of immunosenescence on pulmonary disease. Mediators Inflamm 2015;2015:692546.
9. Ho JC, Chan KN, Hu WH, et al. The effect of aging on nasal mucociliary clearance, beat frequency, and ultrastructure of respiratory cilia. Am J Respir Crit Care Med 2001;163(4):983–8.
10. Svartengren M, Falk R, Philipson K. Long-term clearance from small airways decreases with age. Eur Respir J 2005;26(4):609–15.

11. Hinojosa CA, Akula Suresh Babu R, Rahman MM, et al. Elevated A20 contributes to age-dependent macrophage dysfunction in the lungs. Exp Gerontol 2014;54:58–66.
12. Hinojosa E, Boyd AR, Orihuela CJ. Age-associated inflammation and toll-like receptor dysfunction prime the lungs for pneumococcal pneumonia. J Infect Dis 2009;200(4):546–54.
13. Shivshankar P, Boyd AR, Le Saux CJ, et al. Cellular senescence increases expression of bacterial ligands in the lungs and is positively correlated with increased susceptibility to pneumococcal pneumonia. Aging Cell 2011;10(5): 798–806.
14. Simell B, Vuorela A, Ekstrom N, et al. Aging reduces the functionality of antipneumococcal antibodies and the killing of Streptococcus pneumoniae by neutrophil phagocytosis. Vaccine 2011;29(10):1929–34.
15. Moliva JI, Rajaram MV, Sidiki S, et al. Molecular composition of the alveolar lining fluid in the aging lung. Age 2014;36(3):9633.
16. Kaushik S, Cuervo AM. Proteostasis and aging. Nat Med 2015;21(12):1406–15.
17. Meiners S, Eickelberg O, Konigshoff M. Hallmarks of the ageing lung. Eur Respir J 2015;45(3):807–27.
18. Boyd AR, Shivshankar P, Jiang S, et al. Age-related defects in TLR2 signaling diminish the cytokine response by alveolar macrophages during murine pneumococcal pneumonia. Exp Gerontol 2012;47(7):507–18.
19. Verschoor CP, Johnstone J, Loeb M, et al. Anti-pneumococcal deficits of monocyte-derived macrophages from the advanced-age, frail elderly and related impairments in PI3K-AKT signaling. Hum Immunol 2014;75(12):1192–6.
20. Kline KA, Bowdish DM. Infection in an aging population. Curr Opin Microbiol 2016;29:63–7.
21. Chen MM, Palmer JL, Plackett TP, et al. Age-related differences in the neutrophil response to pulmonary pseudomonas infection. Exp Gerontol 2014;54:42–6.
22. Jackaman C, Radley-Crabb HG, Soffe Z, et al. Targeting macrophages rescues age-related immune deficiencies in C57BL/6J geriatric mice. Aging Cell 2013; 12(3):345–57.
23. Stearns JC, Davidson CJ, McKeon S, et al. Culture and molecular-based profiles show shifts in bacterial communities of the upper respiratory tract that occur with age. ISME J 2015;9(5):1246–59.
24. de Steenhuijsen Piters WA, Huijskens EG, Wyllie AL, et al. Dysbiosis of upper respiratory tract microbiota in elderly pneumonia patients. ISME J 2016;10(1): 97–108.
25. Krone CL, Biesbroek G, Trzcinski K, et al. Respiratory microbiota dynamics following Streptococcus pneumoniae acquisition in young and elderly mice. Infect Immun 2014;82(4):1725–31.
26. Thevaranjan N, Whelan FJ, Puchta A, et al. Streptococcus pneumoniae colonization disrupts the microbial community within the upper respiratory tract of aging mice. Infect Immun 2016;84(4):906–16.
27. Krone CL, Trzcinski K, Zborowski T, et al. Impaired innate mucosal immunity in aged mice permits prolonged Streptococcus pneumoniae colonization. Infect Immun 2013;81(12):4615–25.
28. Whelan FJ, Verschoor CP, Stearns JC, et al. The loss of topography in the microbial communities of the upper respiratory tract in the elderly. Ann Am Thorac Soc 2014;11(4):513–21.
29. Herold S, Mayer K, Lohmeyer J. Acute lung injury: how macrophages orchestrate resolution of inflammation and tissue repair. Front Immunol 2011;2:65.

30. Aggarwal NR, King LS, D'Alessio FR. Diverse macrophage populations mediate acute lung inflammation and resolution. Am J Physiol Lung Cell Mol Physiol 2014;306(8):L709–25.
31. Porcheray F, Viaud S, Rimaniol AC, et al. Macrophage activation switching: an asset for the resolution of inflammation. Clin Exp Immunol 2005;142(3):481–9.
32. Glezeva N, Horgan S, Baugh JA. Monocyte and macrophage subsets along the continuum to heart failure: misguided heroes or targetable villains? J Mol Cell Cardiol 2015;89(Pt B):136–45.
33. Malyshev I, Malyshev Y. Current concept and update of the macrophage plasticity concept: intracellular mechanisms of reprogramming and M3 macrophage "switch" Phenotype. Biomed Res Int 2015;2015:341308.
34. Das A, Sinha M, Datta S, et al. Monocyte and macrophage plasticity in tissue repair and regeneration. Am J Pathol 2015;185(10):2596–606.
35. Mantovani A, Biswas SK, Galdiero MR, et al. Macrophage plasticity and polarization in tissue repair and remodelling. J Pathol 2013;229(2):176–85.
36. Albright JM, Dunn RC, Shults JA, et al. Advanced age alters monocyte and macrophage responses. Antioxid Redox Signal 2016;25(15):805–15.
37. Sica A, Mantovani A. Macrophage plasticity and polarization: in vivo veritas. J Clin Invest 2012;122(3):787–95.
38. Murray PJ, Allen JE, Biswas SK, et al. Macrophage activation and polarization: nomenclature and experimental guidelines. Immunity 2014;41(1):14–20.
39. Ariel A, Maridonneau-Parini I, Rovere-Querini P, et al. Macrophages in inflammation and its resolution. Front Immunol 2012;3:324.
40. Sindrilaru A, Peters T, Wieschalka S, et al. An unrestrained proinflammatory M1 macrophage population induced by iron impairs wound healing in humans and mice. J Clin Invest 2011;121(3):985–97.
41. Shaw AC, Panda A, Joshi SR, et al. Dysregulation of human toll-like receptor function in aging. Ageing Res Rev 2011;10(3):346–53.
42. De Nardo D. Toll-like receptors: activation, signalling and transcriptional modulation. Cytokine 2015;74(2):181–9.
43. Kaparakis M, Philpott DJ, Ferrero RL. Mammalian NLR proteins; discriminating foe from friend. Immunol Cell Biol 2007;85(6):495–502.
44. Renshaw M, Rockwell J, Engleman C, et al. Cutting edge: impaired toll-like receptor expression and function in aging. J Immunol 2002;169(9):4697–701.
45. Boehmer ED, Goral J, Faunce DE, et al. Age-dependent decrease in toll-like receptor 4-mediated proinflammatory cytokine production and mitogen-activated protein kinase expression. J Leukoc Biol 2004;75(2):342–9.
46. Boehmer ED, Meehan MJ, Cutro BT, et al. Aging negatively skews macrophage TLR2- and TLR4-mediated pro-inflammatory responses without affecting the IL-2-stimulated pathway. Mech Ageing Dev 2005;126(12):1305–13.
47. Chelvarajan RL, Collins SM, Van Willigen JM, et al. The unresponsiveness of aged mice to polysaccharide antigens is a result of a defect in macrophage function. J Leukoc Biol 2005;77(4):503–12.
48. Chelvarajan RL, Liu Y, Popa D, et al. Molecular basis of age-associated cytokine dysregulation in LPS-stimulated macrophages. J Leukoc Biol 2006;79(6):1314–27.
49. Liang S, Domon H, Hosur KB, et al. Age-related alterations in innate immune receptor expression and ability of macrophages to respond to pathogen challenge in vitro. Mech Ageing Dev 2009;130(8):538–46.
50. Mahbub S, Deburghgraeve CR, Kovacs EJ. Advanced age impairs macrophage polarization. J Interferon Cytokine Res 2012;32(1):18–26.

51. Arai Y, Martin-Ruiz CM, Takayama M, et al. Inflammation, but not telomere length, predicts successful ageing at extreme old age: a longitudinal study of semi-supercentenarians. EBioMedicine 2015;2(10):1549–58.

52. Swift ME, Kleinman HK, DiPietro LA. Impaired wound repair and delayed angiogenesis in aged mice. Lab Invest 1999;79(12):1479–87.

53. Albright JF, Albright JW. Senescence of natural/innate resistance to infection. Totowa (NY): Humana Press, Inc; 2003.

54. Lynch AM, Murphy KJ, Deighan BF, et al. The impact of glial activation in the aging brain. Aging Dis 2010;1(3):262–78.

55. Linehan E, Dombrowski Y, Snoddy R, et al. Aging impairs peritoneal but not bone marrow-derived macrophage phagocytosis. Aging Cell 2014;13(4): 699–708.

56. Aprahamian T, Takemura Y, Goukassian D, et al. Ageing is associated with diminished apoptotic cell clearance in vivo. Clin Exp Immunol 2008;152(3): 448–55.

57. Arnardottir HH, Dalli J, Colas RA, et al. Aging delays resolution of acute inflammation in mice: reprogramming the host response with novel nano-proresolving medicines. J Immunol 2014;193(8):4235–44.

58. Silva MT. When two is better than one: macrophages and neutrophils work in concert in innate immunity as complementary and cooperative partners of a myeloid phagocyte system. J Leukoc Biol 2010;87(1):93–106.

59. Silva MT, Correia-Neves M. Neutrophils and macrophages: the main partners of phagocyte cell systems. Front Immunol 2012;3:174.

60. Sapey E, Greenwood H, Walton G, et al. Phosphoinositide 3-kinase inhibition restores neutrophil accuracy in the elderly: toward targeted treatments for immunosenescence. Blood 2014;123(2):239–48.

61. Di Lorenzo G, Balistreri CR, Candore G, et al. Granulocyte and natural killer activity in the elderly. Mech Ageing Dev 1999;108(1):25–38.

62. Polignano A, Tortorella C, Venezia A, et al. Age-associated changes of neutrophil responsiveness in a human healthy elderly population. Cytobios 1994; 80(322):145–53.

63. McLaughlin B, O'Malley K, Cotter TG. Age-related differences in granulocyte chemotaxis and degranulation. Clin Sci 1986;70(1):59–62.

64. Antonaci S, Jirillo E, Ventura MT, et al. Non-specific immunity in aging: deficiency of monocyte and polymorphonuclear cell-mediated functions. Mech Ageing Dev 1984;24(3):367–75.

65. Nomellini V, Brubaker AL, Mahbub S, et al. Dysregulation of neutrophil CXCR2 and pulmonary endothelial ICAM-1 promotes age-related pulmonary inflammation. Aging Dis 2012;3(3):234–47.

66. Nomellini V, Faunce DE, Gomez CR, et al. An age-associated increase in pulmonary inflammation after burn injury is abrogated by CXCR2 inhibition. J Leukoc Biol 2008;83(6):1493–501.

67. Brubaker AL, Rendon JL, Ramirez L, et al. Reduced neutrophil chemotaxis and infiltration contributes to delayed resolution of cutaneous wound infection with advanced age. J Immunol 2013;190(4):1746–57.

68. Butcher SK, Chahal H, Nayak L, et al. Senescence in innate immune responses: reduced neutrophil phagocytic capacity and CD16 expression in elderly humans. J Leukoc Biol 2001;70(6):881–6.

69. Butcher SK, Killampalli V, Chahal H, et al. Effect of age on susceptibility to post-traumatic infection in the elderly. Biochem Soc Trans 2003;31(2):449–51.

70. Fulop T Jr, Foris G, Worum I, et al. Age-dependent alterations of Fc gamma receptor-mediated effector functions of human polymorphonuclear leucocytes. Clin Exp Immunol 1985;61(2):425–32.

71. Wenisch C, Patruta S, Daxbock F, et al. Effect of age on human neutrophil function. J Leukoc Biol 2000;67(1):40–5.

72. Amaya RA, Baker CJ, Keitel WA, et al. Healthy elderly people lack neutrophil-mediated functional activity to type V group B *Streptococcus*. J Am Geriatr Soc 2004;52(1):46–50.

73. Butcher S, Chahel H, Lord JM. Review article: ageing and the neutrophil: no appetite for killing? Immunology 2000;100(4):411–6.

74. Alonso-Fernandez P, Puerto M, Mate I, et al. Neutrophils of centenarians show function levels similar to those of young adults. J Am Geriatr Soc 2008;56(12): 2244–51.

75. Esparza B, Sanchez H, Ruiz M, et al. Neutrophil function in elderly persons assessed by flow cytometry. Immunol Invest 1996;25(3):185–90.

76. Dalboni TM, Abe AE, de Oliveira CE, et al. Activation profile of CXCL8-stimulated neutrophils and aging. Cytokine 2013;61(3):716–9.

77. Tortorella C, Ottolenghi A, Pugliese P, et al. Relationship between respiratory burst and adhesiveness capacity in elderly polymorphonuclear cells. Mech Ageing Dev 1993;69(1–2):53–63.

78. Fu YK, Arkins S, Li YM, et al. Reduction in superoxide anion secretion and bactericidal activity of neutrophils from aged rats: reversal by the combination of gamma interferon and growth hormone. Infect Immun 1994;62(1):1–8.

79. Kruger P, Saffarzadeh M, Weber AN, et al. Neutrophils: between host defense, immune modulation, and tissue injury. PLoS Pathog 2015;11(3):e1004651.

80. Tseng CW, Kyme PA, Arruda A, et al. Innate immune dysfunctions in aged mice facilitate the systemic dissemination of methicillin-resistant S. aureus. PLoS One 2012;7(7):e41454.

81. Hazeldine J, Harris P, Chapple IL, et al. Impaired neutrophil extracellular trap formation: a novel defect in the innate immune system of aged individuals. Aging Cell 2014;13(4):690–8.

82. Qian F, Guo X, Wang X, et al. Reduced bioenergetics and toll-like receptor 1 function in human polymorphonuclear leukocytes in aging. Aging (Albany NY) 2014;6(2):131–9.

83. Schroder AK, von der Ohe M, Kolling U, et al. Polymorphonuclear leucocytes selectively produce anti-inflammatory interleukin-1 receptor antagonist and chemokines, but fail to produce pro-inflammatory mediators. Immunology 2006; 119(3):317–27.

84. Fulop T Jr, Fouquet C, Allaire P, et al. Changes in apoptosis of human polymorphonuclear granulocytes with aging. Mech Ageing Dev 1997;96(1–3):15–34.

85. Tortorella C, Simone O, Piazzolla G, et al. Role of phosphoinositide 3-kinase and extracellular signal-regulated kinase pathways in granulocyte macrophage-colony-stimulating factor failure to delay fas-induced neutrophil apoptosis in elderly humans. J Gerontol A Biol Sci Med Sci 2006;61(11):1111–8.

86. Fortin CF, Lesur O, Fulop T Jr. Effects of aging on triggering receptor expressed on myeloid cells (TREM)-1-induced PMN functions. FEBS Lett 2007;581(6): 1173–8.

87. Wessels I, Jansen J, Rink L, et al. Immunosenescence of polymorphonuclear neutrophils. ScientificWorldJournal 2010;10:145–60.

88. Gomez CR, Goral J, Ramirez L, et al. Aberrant acute-phase response in aged interleukin-6 knockout mice. Shock 2006;25(6):581–5.

89. Gomez CR, Hirano S, Cutro BT, et al. Advanced age exacerbates the pulmonary inflammatory response after lipopolysaccharide exposure. Crit Care Med 2007; 35(1):246–51.

90. Gomez CR, Nomellini V, Baila H, et al. Comparison of the effects of aging and IL-6 on the hepatic inflammatory response in two models of systemic injury: scald injury versus I.p. LPS administration. Shock 2009;31(2):178–84.

91. Plowden J, Renshaw-Hoelscher M, Engleman C, et al. Innate immunity in aging: impact on macrophage function. Aging Cell 2004;3(4):161–7.

92. Gomez CR, Karavitis J, Palmer JL, et al. Interleukin-6 contributes to age-related alteration of cytokine production by macrophages. Mediators Inflamm 2010; 2010:475139.

93. Kim KA, Jeong JJ, Yoo SY, et al. Gut microbiota lipopolysaccharide accelerates inflamm-aging in mice. BMC Microbiol 2016;16(1):9.

94. Claesson MJ, Cusack S, O'Sullivan O, et al. Composition, variability, and temporal stability of the intestinal microbiota of the elderly. Proc Natl Acad Sci U S A 2011;108(Suppl 1):4586–91.

95. Claesson MJ, Jeffery IB, Conde S, et al. Gut microbiota composition correlates with diet and health in the elderly. Nature 2012;488(7410):178–84.

96. Langille MG, Meehan CJ, Koenig JE, et al. Microbial shifts in the aging mouse gut. Microbiome 2014;2(1):50.

97. Man AL, Bertelli E, Rentini S, et al. Age-associated modifications of intestinal permeability and innate immunity in human small intestine. Clin Sci 2015; 129(7):515–27.

98. Cesar Machado MC, da Silva FP. Intestinal barrier dysfunction in human pathology and aging. Curr Pharm Des 2016;22(30):4645–50.

99. Pasternak JA, Kent-Dennis C, Van Kessel AG, et al. Claudin-4 undergoes age-dependent change in cellular localization on pig jejunal villous epithelial cells, independent of bacterial colonization. Mediators Inflamm 2015;2015:263629.

100. Valentini L, Ramminger S, Haas V, et al. Small intestinal permeability in older adults. Physiol Rep 2014;2(4):e00281.

101. Mabbott NA. A breakdown in communication? Understanding the effects of aging on the human small intestine epithelium. Clin Sci 2015;129(7):529–31.

102. Mabbott NA, Kobayashi A, Sehgal A, et al. Aging and the mucosal immune system in the intestine. Biogerontology 2015;16(2):133–45.

103. Magnotti LJ, Deitch EA. Burns, bacterial translocation, gut barrier function, and failure. J Burn Care Rehabil 2005;26(5):383–91.

104. Deitch EA. Bacterial translocation or lymphatic drainage of toxic products from the gut: what is important in human beings? Surgery 2002;131(3):241–4.

105. Deitch EA. Gut-origin sepsis: evolution of a concept. Surgeon 2012;10(6):350–6.

106. Ivanov AI. Structure and regulation of intestinal epithelial tight junctions: current concepts and unanswered questions. Adv Exp Med Biol 2012;763:132–48.

107. Ulluwishewa D, Anderson RC, McNabb WC, et al. Regulation of tight junction permeability by intestinal bacteria and dietary components. J Nutr 2011; 141(5):769–76.

108. Hallstrand TS, Hackett TL, Altemeier WA, et al. Airway epithelial regulation of pulmonary immune homeostasis and inflammation. Clin Immunol 2014;151(1): 1–15.

109. Oshima T, Miwa H. Gastrointestinal mucosal barrier function and diseases. J Gastroenterol 2016;51(8):768–78.

110. Dudek SM, Garcia JG. Cytoskeletal regulation of pulmonary vascular permeability. J Appl Physiol (1985) 2001;91(4):1487–500.

111. Odenwald MA, Turner JR. Intestinal permeability defects: is it time to treat? Clin Gastroenterol Hepatol 2013;11(9):1075–83.
112. Turner JR. Molecular basis of epithelial barrier regulation: from basic mechanisms to clinical application. Am J Pathol 2006;169(6):1901–9.
113. Turner JR, Rill BK, Carlson SL, et al. Physiological regulation of epithelial tight junctions is associated with myosin light-chain phosphorylation. Am J Physiol 1997;273(4 Pt 1):C1378–85.
114. Mittal R, Coopersmith CM. Redefining the gut as the motor of critical illness. Trends Mol Med 2014;20(4):214–23.
115. Man AL, Gicheva N, Nicoletti C. The impact of ageing on the intestinal epithelial barrier and immune system. Cell Immunol 2014;289(1–2):112–8.
116. Nicoletti C. Age-associated changes of the intestinal epithelial barrier: local and systemic implications. Expert Rev Gastroenterol Hepatol 2015;9(12):1467–9.
117. Schiffrin EJ, Morley JE, Donnet-Hughes A, et al. The inflammatory status of the elderly: the intestinal contribution. Mutat Res 2010;690(1–2):50–6.
118. Arboleya S, Watkins C, Stanton C, et al. Gut bifidobacteria populations in human health and aging. Front Microbiol 2016;7:1204.
119. Salazar N, Valdes-Varela L, Gonzalez S, et al. Nutrition and the gut microbiome in the elderly. Gut Microbes 2016;8(2):1–16.
120. van Beek AA, Sovran B, Hugenholtz F, et al. Supplementation with lactobacillus plantarum WCFS1 prevents decline of mucus barrier in colon of accelerated aging Ercc1-/Delta7 mice. Front Immunol 2016;7:408.

Lung Diseases of the Elderly: Cellular Mechanisms

Kori Ascher, DO[a], Sharon J. Elliot, PhD[b], Gustavo A. Rubio, MD[b], Marilyn K. Glassberg, MD[a,b,c,*]

KEYWORDS

- Idiopathic pulmonary fibrosis • COPD • Aging • Cellular senescence • Stem cells

KEY POINTS

- Changes in the aging lung result in impaired protective mechanisms that predispose to chronic lung diseases.
- Genomic instability, telomere attrition, and epigenetic alterations are mechanisms that lead to accumulation of genetic errors that result in improper cellular division and development of lung disease.
- Cellular senescence can be induced by cigarette smoking and has been linked to idiopathic pulmonary fibrosis and chronic obstructive pulmonary disease.

AGING LUNG

Aging is the natural process of growing older over a period of time and does not take place uniformly in cells, tissues, or organs.[1] In the lung, aging correlates with the development of chronic lung diseases.[2] Some of the factors that are involved are being characterized, including shorter telomeres, mitochondrial dysfunction, DNA damage, oxidative stress, and changes in markers of apoptosis. An understanding of changes in pulmonary pathophysiology and genomic differentiation in aging lungs may be key to identifying age-related risk factors in the development of lung disease.

INCIDENCE OF LUNG DISEASE INCREASES WITH AGE

As the percentage of persons more than 65 years old increases worldwide (5.87% in 1985, 7.28% in 2005, and 8.28% in 2015[3]), so does the incidence of lung disease.

[a] Division of Pulmonary, Allergy, Critical Care and Sleep Medicine, Department of Medicine, University of Miami Leonard M. Miller School of Medicine, 1600 Northwest 10th Avenue RMSB 7056 (D-60), Miami, FL 33136, USA; [b] DeWitt Daughtry Family Department of Surgery, University of Miami Leonard M. Miller School of Medicine, 1600 NW 10th Avenue, Miami, FL 33136, USA; [c] Division of Pediatric Pulmonology, Department of Pediatrics, University of Miami Leonard M. Miller School of Medicine, 1600 NW 10th Avenue, Miami, FL 33136, USA
* Corresponding author.
E-mail address: mglassbe@med.miami.edu

Clin Geriatr Med 33 (2017) 473–490
http://dx.doi.org/10.1016/j.cger.2017.07.001
0749-0690/17/© 2017 Elsevier Inc. All rights reserved.

Although globally chronic obstructive pulmonary disease (COPD) is reported in 200 per 10,000 patients in individuals less than the age of 45 years, there are 1200 cases reported per 10,000 patients more than the age of 65 years. The predominance of cases in an older age group is also reported in patients with idiopathic pulmonary fibrosis (IPF), in which the incidence increases to about 4 to 17 diagnoses per 10,000 in patients more than the age of 75 years.[4] Overall, there is an almost 5-fold increase in incidence of IPF and COPD related solely to age.[4]

CHANGES IN THE HEALTHY AGING LUNG

There is a natural decline of pulmonary function with aging. Lungs achieve maximum function around 20 to 25 years of age, followed by a steady decline until death.[5] This decline is best shown by the nonlinear decline in forced expiratory volume in 1 second (FEV$_1$) and forced vital capacity (FVC) lung volumes. At approximately 35 to 40 years of age, FEV$_1$ is reduced 25 mL to 30 mL per year. By age 70 years, FEV$_1$ is reduced at a rate of 60 mL per year.[6] Total lung capacity remains constant with advanced age; however, an increase in functional residual capacity and residual volume effectively reduces the vital capacity.[6] Menopause also correlates with a greater decline in FVC than expected with age alone.[7] Differences in men and women regarding sex hormones and their apparent effects on lung function are not yet completely understood.[7] At present, there are limited studies evaluating asymptomatic elderly individuals with radiological imaging and pulmonary function tests; therefore, the full spectrum of the normal aging process remains unknown.

The molecular biology of aging involves multiple mechanisms. Over time, these mechanisms may lose their integrity, resulting in loss of protective strategies. The most studied mechanisms include genomic instability, telomere attrition, epigenetic alterations, proteostasis, nutrient sensing, mitochondrial dysfunction, cell senescence, extracellular matrix (ECM) deregulation, and stem cell exhaustion. Genomic instability may be a result of posttranscriptional changes leading to absent or defective protein products. Usually these defective proteins are eliminated by autophagy. However, if the means by which the cells undergo autophagy is saturated, then abnormal proteins accumulate within the tissue, preventing proper functioning. Telomeres are responsible for protection of chromosomes and assist in genetic stability. With each sequential cell proliferation, telomeres are shortened, and eventually they become too short, resulting in inaccurate cell proliferation. Likewise, stem cell exhaustion and inability to properly regenerate and mitochondrial dysfunction severely limit ATP production, resulting in abnormal cellular functionality.

The Wnt pathway is integral to cell aging.[8] It comprises a group of signal transduction pathways involved in proper regulation of stem cells and progenitor cells, and in maintaining homeostasis during repair from injury. The WNT pathway has been studied in several models of aging organs and is likely a ubiquitous pathway in aging. There are 19 evolutionarily conserved ligands identified.[8–10] The pathway activates β-catenin–dependent (canonical) or β-catenin–independent (noncanonical) pathways.[11] Lung development depends on the WNT pathway for embryogenesis and maintenance of healthy lung tissue. Knockout of this pathway (WNT2 or β-catenin) results in complete agenesis of lungs in mice.[12] Alternatively, when overexpression occurs there is dilation of distal bronchioles, which results in significant respiratory failure.[13] Significantly different levels of specific ligands in this pathway correlate with aging in mice.[14] Aged mouse lungs had different levels of expression of WNT3A at a transcriptional level with altered expressions of target gene Nkd1 compared with young mouse lungs.[15] Similar changes in signaling of WNT pathway with advanced age has been shown in humans.[16] WNT3A expression decreases with advanced age, whereas WNT5A is increased in the aged human lung.[16] Furthermore, there are variations in signaling with advanced age as well as disease-specific patterns identified in different lung diseases.

Reporter mouse models have been used to investigate the healthy aging lung. Of particular interest is the tumor suppressor p19(ARF) (p14 in humans), which is responsible for regulation of cell senescence.[17] Aggregates of p19(ARF) accumulate during aging in mice and are associated with higher compliance of lung tissue. Elimination of p19(ARF) in mice prevented reduced tissue elasticity and other relevant age-related genes found in aging lung tissue, thus leading to improved lung function.[18] Likewise, mitochondrial homeostasis is disrupted, as described by engorged mitochondria of the type II alveolar epithelial cells (AECIIs).[19] There is also dysfunction in autophagy activity described in aging lung fibroblasts.[20]

During homeostasis, AECIIs in aged lung mice models maintain long-term clonal properties with constant proliferation.[21] However, with aging, the proliferation of AECIIs detected by Ki76 staining was markedly slowed compared with young mouse lungs.[21] When challenged with pneumonectomy only, the aged mouse models were unable to increase ECM remodeling compared with young mouse models.[21] The aged mouse model has shown age-related molecular differences that result in impaired response to injury, damage repair, and regeneration of functional tissue.[2]

Regeneration of lung tissue is a multifactorial process. The 3 major known types of respiratory stem cells are airway stem cells, parenchymal stem cells, and alveolar stem cells.[22–25] Airway stem cells from trachea and primary bronchi have the ability to self-renew, proliferate, and differentiate. They respond to insults such as naphthalene injury or viral infection via the Notch pathway to differentiate into club or ciliated cells.[22] Parenchymal stem cells of the bronchoalveolar duct junction can expand in AECIIs and type I alveolar epithelial cells (AECIs) cells after hypoxic injury.[23] In addition, the alveolar stem cells have the ability for clonal expansion and differentiation into either AECIs or AECIIs after injury.[24,25] AECII proliferation depends on, in part, pulmonary capillary endothelial cells (PCEC).[26] When triggered, PCECs upregulate expression of VEGFR2 (vascular endothelial growth factor receptor 2) and FGFR1 (fibroblast growth factor receptor) resulting in proliferation of BASC (bronchi alveolar stem cells), AECII, and PCEC after insult of pneumonectomy.[26] It is hypothesized that the natural decrease in lung function is caused by significantly altered regenerative capabilities of the aforementioned stem cells.

With impaired regulatory mechanisms, there is increased risk for fibrosis after insult[27,28] and decreased ability to restore normal function.[29] Loss of protective repair capability at the cellular level may contribute to age-related lung diseases. The contribution of a dysfunctional aging process and how it relates specifically to COPD, lung cancer, and IPF is discussed later.

CELLULAR HALLMARKS OF PATHOPHYSIOLOGIC AGING
Genomic Instability

Aging has a strong correlation with genetic DNA sequencing defects, likely because of defective DNA repair mechanisms.[30] Accumulation of altered transcription and translational products threaten the inherent properties of normal regeneration.

Genetic susceptibility as a causal factor for obstructive lung disease is not completely understood, although a recent study identified a novel candidate gene that contributes to emphysema susceptibility.[31] In addition, increased breaks in DNA double strands associated with increased levels of oxidative stress have been reported in lung cells of patients with COPD.[32–35] Increased levels of oxidative stress trigger cell death by regulatory protein high mobility group (HMGB1).[36] HMGB1 protein is responsible for autophagy to immunogenic necrosis sensed by oxidative stress.[36] In addition, the canonical WNT signaling pathway is uniquely downregulated in patients with COPD.[37] Decreased signaling can be seen with phenotypic FAM13A gene, another identified COPD susceptibility gene.[37] This initial decreased WNT signaling may be the inciting trigger of COPD development. The full implications of this decreased signaling are not yet well understood, as shown by mouse models of defective DNA repair systems that fail to result in development of lung dysfunction or emphysematous changes.[38]

AGING, LUNG CANCER, AND SMOKING

Cigarette smoke–exposed lung tissue shows alterations in genetic regulation by decreased expression of Werner progeria syndrome protein.[39] Werner progeria protein is a RecQ helicase acting to regulate DNA repair in fibroblasts and epithelial cells in lungs.[39] Although animal knockout mice with DNA repair deficiencies have resulted in significant accumulation of genetic mutation in other organs, the lung has fewer DNA damage aggregates compared with other organs, showing superior restorative properties.[40] Certain single nucleotide polymorphisms hold significant prognostic promise regarding lung cancer progressions as well.

Current evidence suggests that a genetic component may play a role in a subset of patients with IPF. Sputum samples from patients with IPF had microsatellite instability and loss of heterozygosity compared with controls.[41] The microsatellite instability included the gene for transforming growth factor beta (TGF-β), which has been implicated as a profibrotic factor and is responsible for honeycombing in IPF lungs.[42] Other microsatellite defects identified in patients with IPF do not seem to be associated with disease progression or severity.[41,43] Although familial IPF represents a minority of cases, asymptomatic first-degree relatives of patients with IPF were found to have mutations of the regulator of telomere elongation helicase 1 (RTEL1).[44] Heterozygous and homozygous genotypes have been associated with slower and rapid progression of disease, respectively.[44]

Telomere Attrition

Telomeres ensure proper replication of cellular data during division. Telomere dysfunction has previously been studied in several diseases as well as in the aging process. Without the ability to properly proliferate into new healthy cells, there is production of defective cells that contribute to disease progression.

Patients with COPD have consistently shortened telomere lengths in alveolar, endothelial, and smooth muscle cells. Furthermore, the length of telomeres correlates directly with disease severity.[45–48] Telomerase-deficient animal models fail to develop lung emphysema but are more sensitive to cellular alterations in response to cigarette smoke exposure.[48] Mouse models with telomerase deficiency developed pulmonary emphysema only when exposed to cigarette smoke,[48] suggesting that shortened telomeres do not directly cause lung disease but result in an increased sensitivity to noxious stimuli.[49]

Certain tumor cells notoriously generate infinite proliferation by means of repairing naturally shortened telomeres. Prematurely shortened telomeres may pose an early risk for genomic instability and subsequent deregulated proliferation, resulting in neoplasm development.[4]

Telomere attrition also plays a major role in both familial pulmonary fibrosis and IPF.[50,51] Mutations of telomerases significantly reduce their activity level and healthy telomeres are lost at an accelerated rate.[50] Pulmonary fibrosis is the most prevalent clinical feature of underlying mutated telomerases.[50,52–55] Mouse models with deficient telomerase spontaneously develop pulmonary fibrosis.[49] Alternatively, a telomerase activator, GRN 510, was able to inhibit pulmonary fibrosis after bleomycin administration in a murine mouse model.[56]

Epigenetic Alterations

Epigenetic alterations are responsible posttranslation variations of phenotype without a change in the DNA genetic sequence. These alterations include DNA or histone methylation, acetylation, phosphorylation, ubiquitinylation, sumoylation, ribosylation, citrullination, RNA spicing, and noncoding RNAs (microRNAs [miRNAs]). Many cellular processes are influenced by epigenetic changes, including gene expression, cellular differentiation, genomic imprinting, and embryogenesis.[57]

These naturally occurring variations to DNA and RNA have been a major area of study for aging in various organs.[8] Age-related DNA methylation pattern changes have been termed the epigenetic clock.[5] Exogenous irritants such as cigarette smoke have been found to affect DNA methylation patterns. Lung function and severity of disease also correlate with DNA methylation.[58] Compared with control lungs, there are unique identifiable epigenetic alterations of histones and messenger RNA (mRNA) in COPD lungs.[59]

Epigenetic disruptions are abundant in tumor cells.[60] Expression of various changes is vast and certain patterns are associated with worse prognosis.[61] As stated previously, exposure to cigarette smoke results in epigenetic alterations that may predispose to pulmonary cancers. However, no specific pattern has been identified as oncogenic.[62,63]

MiRNAs alter gene expression posttranscriptionally. Altered miRNA expression profiles have been reported in asthma,[64] COPD,[65] cystic fibrosis,[66] and IPF[67] (**Tables 1** and **2**), as well as lung cancer.[68,69] These alterations have been noted in isolated lung tissue, sputum, bronchoalveolar lavage fluids, and peripheral blood or serum. The roles of specific miRNAs in the pathogenesis of COPD and pulmonary fibrosis

Table 1
MicroRNAs dysregulated in idiopathic pulmonary fibrosis

	Upregulated/Downregulated	Reference
Profibrotic		
miR-21	Up	76
miR-96	Up	72
miR-155	Up	77
miR-154	Up	78
Antifibrotic		
miR-29	Down	67
let-7d	Down	79
miR-30	Down	67
miR-200	Down	59
miR-326	Down	80
miR-26	Down	81

Table 2 Targets of selected microRNAs	
MiRNAs Targeting Insulin/IGF[82–84]	MiRNAs Targeting Sirt1[85]
miR-1	miR-34a
miR-206	miR-449
miR-21	miR-181 a/b
miR-122	miR-9
miR-375	miR-195
	miR-22
	miR-200a

Abbreviation: IGF, insulinlike growth factor.

have been extensively studied in both human tissues and experimental rodent models.[70–72] For example, decreased expression of miR-17-92 in IPF lungs leads to increased DNA methylase (DNMT-1).[73] As mentioned previously, altered methylation patterns have significant effects on specific genes that promote pulmonary fibrosis.[74] In addition, acetylation may also be pertinent, with manipulation of histone acetylation inhibiting bleomycin-induced pulmonary fibrosis in mice.[75]

Dysregulated proteostasis

Proteostasis refers to the controlled regulation of cellular protein synthesis, folding, trafficking, and degradation. Dysregulation may result in nonfunctioning proteins, mis-signaling proteins, or aggregation of improperly degraded proteins.

COPD has been associated with dysregulated proteostasis. Exposure to irritants, such as cigarette smoke, creates alterations to the ubiquitin-proteasomal degradation system that identify proteins for premature degradation.[86] These alterations include varying degrees of oxidative stress or misfolded proteins. Autophagy or proteasome activity predominates regarding protein degradation; however, in patients with COPD, there is reduced proteasome activity with increased autophagy activity compared with healthy individuals.[87,88] The degree of proteasome activity reduction correlates with severity of lung dysfunction.[87] In addition, there are selected autophagy pathways that have been associated with mediating ciliary dysfunction in patients with COPD.[89]

Tumors are associated with alterations in proteostasis that promote cellular survival, which is accomplished mostly via altered signaling of endoplasmic reticulum (ER) and autophagy.[4] It has been suggested that tumor cells are able to reprogram signaling of ER and autophagy to promote self-survival.[90,91]

Proteostasis also has a seemingly large role in IPF. More specifically, proteasome inhibitors suppress pulmonary fibrosis in bleomycin-treated mouse models.[92] Aberrant activation of the mammalian target of rapamycin (mTor) pathway resulting in defective autophagy has been reported in IPF.[93–95] Particularly in familial IPF, there are defective secretory proteins caused by abnormal ER function. Abnormal proteins cannot exit the ER and therefore accumulate within the cell resulting in unfolded protein response.[96] Similar ER stress associated with unfolded protein response has been reported in AECIIs in patients with IPF.[97] ER stress with resultant unfolded protein response has been a topic of interest in fibrosis. Murine gamma herpesvirus infection in epithelial cells induced ER stress and an unfolded protein response.[98] Furthermore, those murine mice infected with murine gamma herpesvirus developed clinical features that paralleled those of IPF.[27]

Nutrient Sensing

Cellular growth requires nutrition and accurate signaling of nutrient availability. It is achieved by the evolutionary conserved insulinlike growth factor (IGF)-1/AKT (protein kinase B)/mTOR (mechanistic target of rapamycin) axis,[99,100] which plays a major role in COPD, lung cancer, and IPF. Caloric restriction suppresses this axis, promoting cell life span.[89,101] SIRT3 (Sirtuin 3), a mitochondrial deacetylase, inhibits acetylation of mitochondrial proteins.[102,103] SIRT3 is stimulated by caloric restriction, resulting in lower levels of inflammation via the interleukin-1beta (IL-1β) pathway.[104] Once acetylation occurs, there is activation of inflammation with increased IL-1β levels.[104] Basal levels of chronic inflammation have been linked to the noncommunicative chronic lung diseases that are discussed in this article.

Emphysematous lungs can be produced in animal models by manipulating the IGF-1/AKT/mTOR axis. Changes to the IGF-1/AKT/mTOR axis to limit or increase activity in animal mouse models exposed to cigarette smoke had either development of emphysematous lungs or resistance to cigarette smoke–induced emphysema, respectively.[105] As stated earlier, mTOR signaling is closely associated with autophagy.[105] The increase in autophagy noted at baseline in bronchial epithelial cells isolated from COPD lungs[106] may alter this pathway's regulation of inflammation and life cycle control. Under normal conditions these pathways suppress autophagy and promote apoptosis by means of forkhead box O (FOXO) activation.[107] Patients with COPD have lower levels of FOXO, whereas FOXO knockout mice models have more severe emphysema after smoke exposure.[108] Cigarette smoke–induced inhibition of SIRT6 has been shown to activate the IGF-1/AKT/mTOR pathway and inhibit autophagy[109] in human bronchial epithelial cells.

Viability of tumor cells also depends on prolonged proliferation, which is obtained by perpetual activation of the IGF-1/AKT/mTOR axis via various molecular pathways.[4] This topic is well described in a recent review article.[110]

There is a decreased level of autophagy activity and increased expression of IGF in IPF.[111] IGF-1 overexpression leads to pulmonary fibrosis in animal models; alternatively, when suppressed, there is protection against bleomycin-induced pulmonary fibrosis.[112] Inhibition of mTOR with rapamycin has protective properties on TGF-β–induced fibrotic mice.[113] Likewise, activated mTOR enhanced IPF fibroblast apoptosis resistance.[20] Under starvation conditions, there is more dysfunctional autophagy and persistent activation of the mTOR pathway.[5,20] Furthermore, under starvation conditions, young healthy mouse models failed to show the same changes in autophagy and mTOR pathway as were seen in the old mice and IPF models.[5]

Mitochondrial Dysfunction

Enlarged defective mitochondria are found at increased frequency in aged AECIIs.[19] This development is likely related to the abnormal respiratory capacity (loss of mitochondrial cristae) and increased mitochondrial radical oxidative stress.[19,114] In addition, aged mitochondria produce more oxidative stress.[115,116] Abnormal mitochondria accumulate in several differentiated tissue types with aging.[117,118] This accumulation may in part be caused by decreased expression of mitochondrial SIRT3, an antioxidant, found in healthy aged mice.[114,119] PTEN (phosphatidylinositol phosphate 3'-phosphatase)–induced putative kinase 1 (PINK1), another important mitochondrial regulator of proper clearance of defective mitochondria, is found in decreased expression with advanced age.[19] For this reason, the pathways maintaining mitochondrial integrity have been of particular interest regarding aging and lung disease.

Cigarette smoke induces changes in mitochondrial structure and function. Recent data suggest a role of aberrant mitochondrial function or regulation in the pathogenesis of COPD, as outlined in the excellent review by Kang and colleagues.[120]

Mitochondrial dysfunction promotes tumor growth by increased reactive oxygen species (ROS) production.[121] Increased ROS decreases apoptosis, leading to tumorigenesis; however, it has not yet been identified as an initial triggering factor for lung cancer development.[122] Retrograde signaling (signal from mitochondria to nucleus) dysregulation may also lead to age-related lung diseases.[123]

The role of dysfunctional mitochondria in IPF pathogenesis is becoming more apparent. Lung fibrosis can be replicated when aged AECIIs manipulate the mitochondrial communication signals.[5] The defective mitochondria in both IPF and AECIIs are caused by decreased PINK1 expression.[5] PINK1 knockout mice induced apoptosis and increased TGF-β expression, causing lung fibrosis.[19] Mitochondrial SIRT3 deficiency, briefly mentioned earlier, has been associated with degree of severity of pulmonary fibrosis.[124]

Cellular Senescence

Senescence is the ability of a cell to have programmed cell cycle arrest. Conditions such as stress or inflammation may trigger a cell to enter this state. Senescence allows cells to evade apoptosis.[29] Increased senescence has been linked to IPF and COPD disease processes.[125] It has been proposed that the increase is a direct result of different WNT ligand activation.[115,126] Senescence in the aging lung model results in a cellular state that increases production of inflammatory mediators and growth factors, including cytokines, chemokines, and proteases.[74,127] Importantly, senescence can be induced by cigarette smoke exposure.[39] Furthermore, progression of COPD in lung tissue has been associated with increased senescence of endothelial and parenchymal cells.[126] This increased senescence may in part be caused by increased signaling of the WNT pathway in parallel with decreased levels of the antiaging protein Klotho.[126] Klotho null mice reveal an increased vulnerability and susceptibility to injury in lung tissue induced by cigarette smoke, as shown by development of emphysema.[128] More recent data show that Klotho treatment of alveolar macrophages can attenuate cigarette smoke–induced autophagy and inhibit AKT/IGF pathway signaling.[129]

Cell cycle arrest plays a major role in tumor cells. Senescence acts as a protective strategy to prevent uncontrolled proliferation in damaged, cigarette smoke–induced lung cells. Loss of this protective strategy marks the beginning of tumorigenesis with uncontrolled growth.[130]

Increased cellular senescence has been described as one of the key features of IPF, as identified by staining for β-gal and p21 expression.[131,132] IPF telomere dysfunction, as previously discussed, effectively induces cellular senescence in IPF.[5] Similarly, bleomycin-induced fibrosis mouse models showed resistance to fibrosis when there was reduced senescence detected in bone marrow stem cells[133] and showed that normalization of the imbalance of Nox4 (which mediates production of ROS) and Nrf2 (antioxidant transcription factor) can reverse senescence and apoptosis. Stress-induced senescence has a self-limiting course in young fibroblasts, a phenomenon that is lost in aged fibroblasts.[29]

Stem Cell Exhaustion

Stem cells characteristically maintain the ability to differentiate into any cell type, including different cells with preprogramed life cycles (ie, erythrocyte vs platelet vs lymphocyte). The constant need to replace a particular cell type results in stem cell fatigue, inhibiting their ability to properly differentiate. The lung is a slow turnover organ[134]; however, cellular damage requiring tissue repair increases turnover demand for stem cells. Within the healthy conducting system, pools of stem cells have been identified as well as basal cells with progenitor capability within the airway.[135] Furthermore, AECIIs differentiate into AECIs, showing intrinsic stem cell functionality.[24] Stem cell exhaustion and loss of lung tissue ability to self-repair may represent the fundamental cause of age-related lung disease. These mechanisms are being actively investigated for therapeutic (possibly curative) management of age-related lung disease, and this is especially true for IPF.

Smoke exposure causes direct damage to AECIIs, therefore their stem cell capability to regenerate is lost and healthy cells cannot replace the damaged cells.[136] In addition, the endothelial progenitor cells that maintain some ability to function have defective DNA that compromises cell differentiation.[137] Basal cells and AECIIs from patients with COPD have limited regenerative properties with inability to fully differentiate into epithelium.[137,138] Furthermore, bone marrow–derived stem cells from patients with COPD have impaired ability to regenerate.[138] WNT ligands interfere with alveolar epithelial cell differentiation capability, leading to direct development of emphysema.[139]

Inability to proliferate and regenerate may be a protective property to prevent lung cancer. Stem cells with defective DNA proliferate damaged cells that can promote tumor cells, as has been described in non–small cell lung cancer.[121,140] There is growing evidence that there are increased quantity of mesenchymal stem cells (MSCs) detected in fibrotic lung. However, when lung MSCs (LMSCs) isolated from young mice were compared with LMSCs from older mice, there was reduced mRNA expression of retinoic acid (*Aldh1a3, Rbp4*), Fgf/Wnt (*Fgfr1, Sfrp1, Wnt2,* and *Ctnnb1*), and elastogenesis (*Col1a1, Eln, Fbn1,* and *Sdc2*) pathway genes. Isolated LMSCs from older mice also showed fewer colony-forming units (−67%) and less growth potential (−60% by day 7), ALDH activity (−49%), and telomerase activity (−47%). Therefore, age is associated with declining proliferative potential and regenerative functions of LMSCs in the lung.[21]

Similar to COPD, stem cells from patients with IPF show reduced ability to properly differentiate during lung tissue repair. In contrast with COPD, there is evidence of hyperplastic alveolar epithelial cells contributing to IPF disease process.[141] AECIIs also have impaired regenerative capacity in IPF.[142] There are presently several ongoing clinical trials using stem cells as therapeutic agents to replace this loss of self-protection, with promising results showing the safety of this therapy.[143–146]

Extracellular Matrix Dysfunction

The ECM is an organ-unique structure undergoing constant remodeling. Homeostatic regulation of this structure is crucial for proper organ development. ECM maintenance is a balance between collagen deposition and degradation by metalloproteinases (MMPs). Integrity of ECM maintains physical support for tissue integrity, elasticity, as well as overall tissue homeostasis. Age-related changes to the delicate balance of proteinase/antiproteinase of the ECM significantly increase susceptibility to COPD, lung cancer, and IPF.[1,147,148] The ability of cells to produce and secrete components of the ECM changes with age.[149]

Dysregulated MMPs have been found in COPD lung cells. The balance is favored toward increased proteinase activity resulting in loss of alveolar septae and emphysematous formation.[150,151] Reduced expression of specific ECM glycoprotein fibulin-4 results in spontaneous development of emphysema in mouse models.[152]

Dysregulation of the ECM has also been described within lung cancer cells.[121] ECM promotes tumor growth, in part, by neoangiogenesis.[153] The ECM molecules fibronectin and integrin are involved in metastatic lung cancer growth.[154] Overexpression of collagen IV promotes lung cancer cell growth by evading apoptosis.[155] In other organs, high levels of MMPs correlate with poor prognosis, whereas lower levels of protease inhibitors correlate with better prognosis.[156] In small cell lung cancer, chemotherapy resistance is related to abnormally extensive ECM promoting survival.[157]

Abnormal ECM has also been implicated as causing IPF disease progression. ECM from patients with IPF has increased ECM production in not only IPF fibroblasts but in non-IPF fibroblasts as well.[158] Because of the profibrotic properties of ECM, studies investigating interventions targeting MMPs as therapeutic agents are ongoing. Fibrosis can be induced with decreased expression of the genetic regulator of ECM, Twist1.[159] Decreased Twist1 expression increases inflammatory markers in IPF models. Furthermore, deletion of Twist1 accelerates the fibrotic process.[159] Older fibroblast cells and AECIIs secrete ECM that promotes myofibroblast differentiation, creating a positive feedback loop that promotes this profibrotic process.[160,161]

SUMMARY

Natural lung aging is characterized by molecular and cellular changes in multiple lung cell populations. These changes include shorter telomeres, increased expression of cellular senescence markers, increased DNA damage, oxidative stress, apoptosis, and stem cell exhaustion. Aging, combined with the loss of protective repair processes, correlates with the development and incidence of chronic respiratory diseases, including idiopathic pulmonary fibrosis and chronic obstructive pulmonary disease. Ultimately, it is the interplay of age-related changes in biology and the subsequent responses to environmental exposures that largely define the physiology and clinical course of the aging lung.

REFERENCES

1. Jones OR, Scheuerlein A, Salguero-Gomez R, et al. Diversity of ageing across the tree of life. Nature 2014;505(7482):169–73.
2. Navarro S, Driscoll B. Regeneration of the aging lung: a mini-review. Gerontology 2017;63(3):270–80.
3. Bank TW. Population ages 65 and above (% of total). 2015; Available at: http://data.worldbank.org/indicator/SP.POP.65UP.TO.ZS?locations=US. Accessed June 8, 2017.
4. Meiners S, Eickelberg O, Konigshoff M. Hallmarks of the ageing lung. Eur Respir J 2015;45(3):807–27.
5. Mora AL, Bueno M, Rojas M. Mitochondria in the spotlight of aging and idiopathic pulmonary fibrosis. J Clin Invest 2017;127(2):405–14.
6. Sharma G, Goodwin J. Effect of aging on respiratory system physiology and immunology. Clin Interv Aging 2006;1(3):253–60.
7. Triebner K, Matulonga B, Johannessen A, et al. Menopause is associated with accelerated lung function decline. Am J Respir Crit Care Med 2017;195(8):1058–65.
8. Lopez-Otin C, Blasco MA, Partridge L, et al. The hallmarks of aging. Cell 2013;153(6):1194–217.
9. Konigshoff M, Eickelberg O. WNT signaling in lung disease: a failure or a regeneration signal? Am J Respir Cell Mol Biol 2010;42(1):21–31.
10. Thannickal VJ, Murthy M, Balch WE, et al. Blue journal conference. Aging and susceptibility to lung disease. Am J Respir Crit Care Med 2015;191(3):261–9.

11. Lehmann M, Baarsma HA, Konigshoff M. WNT signaling in lung aging and disease. Ann Am Thorac Soc 2016;13(Suppl 5):S411–6.
12. Goss AM, Tian Y, Tsukiyama T, et al. Wnt2/2b and beta-catenin signaling are necessary and sufficient to specify lung progenitors in the foregut. Dev Cell 2009;17(2):290–8.
13. Li C, Hu L, Xiao J, et al. Wnt5a regulates Shh and Fgf10 signaling during lung development. Dev Biol 2005;287(1):86–97.
14. Hofmann JW, McBryan T, Adams PD, et al. The effects of aging on the expression of Wnt pathway genes in mouse tissues. Age (Dordr) 2014;36(3):9618.
15. Kneidinger N, Yildirim AO, Callegari J, et al. Activation of the WNT/beta-catenin pathway attenuates experimental emphysema. Am J Respir Crit Care Med 2011;183(6):723–33.
16. Kovacs T, Csongei V, Feller D, et al. Alteration in the Wnt microenvironment directly regulates molecular events leading to pulmonary senescence. Aging Cell 2014;13(5):838–49.
17. Ben-Porath I, Weinberg RA. The signals and pathways activating cellular senescence. Int J Biochem Cell Biol 2005;37(5):961–76.
18. Hashimoto M, Asai A, Kawagishi H, et al. Elimination of p19ARF-expressing cells enhances pulmonary function in mice. JCI Insight 2016;1(12):e87732.
19. Bueno M, Lai YC, Romero Y, et al. PINK1 deficiency impairs mitochondrial homeostasis and promotes lung fibrosis. J Clin Invest 2015;125(2):521–38.
20. Romero Y, Bueno M, Ramirez R, et al. mTORC1 activation decreases autophagy in aging and idiopathic pulmonary fibrosis and contributes to apoptosis resistance in IPF fibroblasts. Aging Cell 2016. [Epub ahead of print].
21. Paxson JA, Gruntman AM, Davis AM, et al. Age dependence of lung mesenchymal stromal cell dynamics following pneumonectomy. Stem Cells Dev 2013;22(24):3214–25.
22. Song H, Yao E, Lin C, et al. Functional characterization of pulmonary neuroendocrine cells in lung development, injury, and tumorigenesis. Proc Natl Acad Sci U S A 2012;109(43):17531–6.
23. Rawlins EL, Okubo T, Xue Y, et al. The role of Scgb1a1+ Clara cells in the long-term maintenance and repair of lung airway, but not alveolar, epithelium. Cell Stem Cell 2009;4(6):525–34.
24. Barkauskas CE, Cronce MJ, Rackley CR, et al. Type 2 alveolar cells are stem cells in adult lung. J Clin Invest 2013;123(7):3025–36.
25. Jain R, Barkauskas CE, Takeda N, et al. Plasticity of Hopx(+) type I alveolar cells to regenerate type II cells in the lung. Nat Commun 2015;6:6727.
26. Ding BS, Nolan DJ, Guo P, et al. Endothelial-derived angiocrine signals induce and sustain regenerative lung alveolarization. Cell 2011;147(3):539–53.
27. Torres-Gonzalez E, Bueno M, Tanaka A, et al. Role of endoplasmic reticulum stress in age-related susceptibility to lung fibrosis. Am J Respir Cell Mol Biol 2012;46(6):748–56.
28. Sueblinvong V, Neujahr DC, Mills ST, et al. Predisposition for disrepair in the aged lung. Am J Med Sci 2012;344(1):41–51.
29. Hecker L, Logsdon NJ, Kurundkar D, et al. Reversal of persistent fibrosis in aging by targeting Nox4-Nrf2 redox imbalance. Sci Transl Med 2014;6(231):231ra247.
30. Moskalev AA, Shaposhnikov MV, Plyusnina EN, et al. The role of DNA damage and repair in aging through the prism of Koch-like criteria. Ageing Res Rev 2013;12(2):661–84.

31. Radder JE, Zhang Y, Gregory AD, et al. Extreme trait whole genome sequencing identifies PTPRO as a novel candidate gene in emphysema with severe airflow obstruction. Am J Respir Crit Care Med 2017;196(2):159–71.
32. Aoshiba K, Zhou F, Tsuji T, et al. DNA damage as a molecular link in the pathogenesis of COPD in smokers. Eur Respir J 2012;39(6):1368–76.
33. Makris D, Tzanakis N, Damianaki A, et al. Microsatellite DNA instability and COPD exacerbations. Eur Respir J 2008;32(3):612–8.
34. Tzortzaki EG, Dimakou K, Neofytou E, et al. Oxidative DNA damage and somatic mutations: a link to the molecular pathogenesis of chronic inflammatory airway diseases. Chest 2012;141(5):1243–50.
35. Caramori G, Adcock IM, Casolari P, et al. Unbalanced oxidant-induced DNA damage and repair in COPD: a link towards lung cancer. Thorax 2011;66(6):521–7.
36. Munoz-Espin D, Serrano M. Cellular senescence: from physiology to pathology. Nat Rev Mol Cell Biol 2014;15(7):482–96.
37. Jin Z, Chung JW, Mei W, et al. Regulation of nuclear-cytoplasmic shuttling and function of Family with sequence similarity 13, member A (Fam13a), by B56-containing PP2As and Akt. Mol Biol Cell 2015;26(6):1160–73.
38. German J. Bloom's syndrome. I. Genetical and clinical observations in the first twenty-seven patients. Am J Hum Genet 1969;21(2):196–227.
39. Nyunoya T, Monick MM, Klingelhutz AL, et al. Cigarette smoke induces cellular senescence via Werner's syndrome protein down-regulation. Am J Respir Crit Care Med 2009;179(4):279–87.
40. Uehara Y, Ikehata H, Furuya M, et al. XPC is involved in genome maintenance through multiple pathways in different tissues. Mutat Res 2009;670(1–2):24–31.
41. Vassilakis DA, Sourvinos G, Spandidos DA, et al. Frequent genetic alterations at the microsatellite level in cytologic sputum samples of patients with idiopathic pulmonary fibrosis. Am J Respir Crit Care Med 2000;162(3 Pt 1):1115–9.
42. Mori M, Kida H, Morishita H, et al. Microsatellite instability in transforming growth factor-beta 1 type II receptor gene in alveolar lining epithelial cells of idiopathic pulmonary fibrosis. Am J Respir Cell Mol Biol 2001;24(4):398–404.
43. Samara K, Zervou M, Siafakas NM, et al. Microsatellite DNA instability in benign lung diseases. Respir Med 2006;100(2):202–11.
44. Cogan JD, Kropski JA, Zhao M, et al. Rare variants in RTEL1 are associated with familial interstitial pneumonia. Am J Respir Crit Care Med 2015;191(6):646–55.
45. Amsellem V, Gary-Bobo G, Marcos E, et al. Telomere dysfunction causes sustained inflammation in chronic obstructive pulmonary disease. Am J Respir Crit Care Med 2011;184(12):1358–66.
46. Morla M, Busquets X, Pons J, et al. Telomere shortening in smokers with and without COPD. Eur Respir J 2006;27(3):525–8.
47. Tsuji T, Aoshiba K, Nagai A. Cigarette smoke induces senescence in alveolar epithelial cells. Am J Respir Cell Mol Biol 2004;31(6):643–9.
48. Alder JK, Guo N, Kembou F, et al. Telomere length is a determinant of emphysema susceptibility. Am J Respir Crit Care Med 2011;184(8):904–12.
49. Povedano JM, Martinez P, Flores JM, et al. Mice with pulmonary fibrosis driven by telomere dysfunction. Cell Rep 2015;12(2):286–99.
50. Alder JK, Chen JJ, Lancaster L, et al. Short telomeres are a risk factor for idiopathic pulmonary fibrosis. Proc Natl Acad Sci U S A 2008;105(35):13051–6.
51. Armanios M, Blackburn EH. The telomere syndromes. Nat Rev Genet 2012;13(10):693–704.

52. Armanios MY, Chen JJ, Cogan JD, et al. Telomerase mutations in families with idiopathic pulmonary fibrosis. N Engl J Med 2007;356(13):1317–26.
53. Cronkhite JT, Xing C, Raghu G, et al. Telomere shortening in familial and sporadic pulmonary fibrosis. Am J Respir Crit Care Med 2008;178(7):729–37.
54. Tsakiri KD, Cronkhite JT, Kuan PJ, et al. Adult-onset pulmonary fibrosis caused by mutations in telomerase. Proc Natl Acad Sci U S A 2007;104(18):7552–7.
55. Fingerlin TE, Murphy E, Zhang W, et al. Genome-wide association study identifies multiple susceptibility loci for pulmonary fibrosis. Nat Genet 2013;45(6): 613–20.
56. Le Saux CJ, Davy P, Brampton C, et al. A novel telomerase activator suppresses lung damage in a murine model of idiopathic pulmonary fibrosis. PLoS One 2013;8(3):e58423.
57. Codd V, Nelson CP, Albrecht E, et al. Identification of seven loci affecting mean telomere length and their association with disease. Nat Genet 2013;45(4):422–7, 427.e1-2.
58. Qiu W, Baccarelli A, Carey VJ, et al. Variable DNA methylation is associated with chronic obstructive pulmonary disease and lung function. Am J Respir Crit Care Med 2012;185(4):373–81.
59. Yang S, Banerjee S, de Freitas A, et al. Participation of miR-200 in pulmonary fibrosis. Am J Pathol 2012;180(2):484–93.
60. Baylin SB, Jones PA. A decade of exploring the cancer epigenome - biological and translational implications. Nat Rev Cancer 2011;11(10):726–34.
61. You JS, Jones PA. Cancer genetics and epigenetics: two sides of the same coin? Cancer Cell 2012;22(1):9–20.
62. Jakopovic M, Thomas A, Balasubramaniam S, et al. Targeting the epigenome in lung cancer: expanding approaches to epigenetic therapy. Front Oncol 2013;3:261.
63. Smith LT, Lin M, Brena RM, et al. Epigenetic regulation of the tumor suppressor gene TCF21 on 6q23-q24 in lung and head and neck cancer. Proc Natl Acad Sci U S A 2006;103(4):982–7.
64. Tay HL, Plank M, Collison A, et al. MicroRNA: potential biomarkers and therapeutic targets for allergic asthma? Ann Med 2014;46(8):633–9.
65. De Smet EG, Mestdagh P, Vandesompele J, et al. Non-coding RNAs in the pathogenesis of COPD. Thorax 2015;70(8):782–91.
66. Sonneville F, Ruffin M, Guillot L, et al. New insights about miRNAs in cystic fibrosis. Am J Pathol 2015;185(4):897–908.
67. Pandit KV, Milosevic J, Kaminski N. MicroRNAs in idiopathic pulmonary fibrosis. Transl Res 2011;157(4):191–9.
68. Lin PY, Yu SL, Yang PC. MicroRNA in lung cancer. Br J Cancer 2010;103(8): 1144–8.
69. Rusek AM, Abba M, Eljaszewicz A, et al. MicroRNA modulators of epigenetic regulation, the tumor microenvironment and the immune system in lung cancer. Mol Cancer 2015;14:34.
70. Yang G, Yang L, Wang W, et al. Discovery and validation of extracellular/circulating microRNAs during idiopathic pulmonary fibrosis disease progression. Gene 2015;562(1):138–44.
71. Pandit KV, Milosevic J. MicroRNA regulatory networks in idiopathic pulmonary fibrosis. Biochem Cell Biol 2015;93(2):129–37.
72. Nho RS. Alteration of aging-dependent microRNAs in idiopathic pulmonary fibrosis. Drug Dev Res 2015;76(7):343–53.

73. Dakhlallah D, Batte K, Wang Y, et al. Epigenetic regulation of miR-17~92 contributes to the pathogenesis of pulmonary fibrosis. Am J Respir Crit Care Med 2013;187(4):397–405.

74. Sanders YY, Ambalavanan N, Halloran B, et al. Altered DNA methylation profile in idiopathic pulmonary fibrosis. Am J Respir Crit Care Med 2012;186(6): 525–35.

75. Sanders YY, Hagood JS, Liu H, et al. Histone deacetylase inhibition promotes fibroblast apoptosis and ameliorates pulmonary fibrosis in mice. Eur Respir J 2014;43(5):1448–58.

76. Liu G, Friggeri A, Yang Y, et al. miR-21 mediates fibrogenic activation of pulmonary fibroblasts and lung fibrosis. J Exp Med 2010;207(8):1589–97.

77. Pottier N, Maurin T, Chevalier B, et al. Identification of keratinocyte growth factor as a target of microRNA-155 in lung fibroblasts: implication in epithelial-mesenchymal interactions. PLoS One 2009;4(8):e6718.

78. Milosevic J, Pandit K, Magister M, et al. Profibrotic role of miR-154 in pulmonary fibrosis. Am J Respir Cell Mol Biol 2012;47(6):879–87.

79. Pandit KV, Corcoran D, Yousef H, et al. Inhibition and role of let-7d in idiopathic pulmonary fibrosis. Am J Respir Crit Care Med 2010;182(2):220–9.

80. Das S, Kumar M, Negi V, et al. MicroRNA-326 regulates profibrotic functions of transforming growth factor-beta in pulmonary fibrosis. Am J Respir Cell Mol Biol 2014;50(5):882–92.

81. Liang H, Gu Y, Li T, et al. Integrated analyses identify the involvement of microRNA-26a in epithelial-mesenchymal transition during idiopathic pulmonary fibrosis. Cell Death Dis 2014;5:e1238.

82. Jung HJ, Suh Y. MicroRNA in aging: from discovery to biology. Curr Genomics 2012;13(7):548–57.

83. Wang XH, Qian RZ, Zhang W, et al. MicroRNA-320 expression in myocardial microvascular endothelial cells and its relationship with insulin-like growth factor-1 in type 2 diabetic rats. Clin Exp Pharmacol Physiol 2009;36(2):181–8.

84. Shan ZX, Lin QX, Fu YH, et al. Upregulated expression of miR-1/miR-206 in a rat model of myocardial infarction. Biochem Biophys Res Commun 2009;381(4): 597–601.

85. Lize M, Klimke A, Dobbelstein M. MicroRNA-449 in cell fate determination. Cell Cycle 2011;10(17):2874–82.

86. Meiners S, Eickelberg O. What shall we do with the damaged proteins in lung disease? Ask the proteasome! Eur Respir J 2012;40(5):1260–8.

87. Chen ZH, Lam HC, Jin Y, et al. Autophagy protein microtubule-associated protein 1 light chain-3B (LC3B) activates extrinsic apoptosis during cigarette smoke-induced emphysema. Proc Natl Acad Sci U S A 2010;107(44):18880–5.

88. Ryter SW, Chen ZH, Kim HP, et al. Autophagy in chronic obstructive pulmonary disease: homeostatic or pathogenic mechanism? Autophagy 2009;5(2):235–7.

89. Cheng CW, Adams GB, Perin L, et al. Prolonged fasting reduces IGF-1/PKA to promote hematopoietic-stem-cell-based regeneration and reverse immunosuppression. Cell Stem Cell 2014;14(6):810–23.

90. Marcinak SJ, Ron D. The unfolded protein response in lung disease. Proc Am Thorac Soc 2010;7(6):356–62.

91. Mah LY, Ryan KM. Autophagy and cancer. Cold Spring Harb Perspect Biol 2012; 4(1):a008821.

92. Mutlu GM, Budinger GR, Wu M, et al. Proteasomal inhibition after injury prevents fibrosis by modulating TGF-beta(1) signalling. Thorax 2012;67(2):139–46.

93. Patel AS, Lin L, Geyer A, et al. Autophagy in idiopathic pulmonary fibrosis. PLoS One 2012;7(7):e41394.

94. Araya J, Kojima J, Takasaka N, et al. Insufficient autophagy in idiopathic pulmonary fibrosis. Am J Physiol Lung Cell Mol Physiol 2013;304(1):L56–69.

95. Ricci A, Cherubini E, Scozzi D, et al. Decreased expression of autophagic beclin 1 protein in idiopathic pulmonary fibrosis fibroblasts. J Cell Physiol 2013; 228(7):1516–24.

96. Tanjore H, Blackwell TS, Lawson WE. Emerging evidence for endoplasmic reticulum stress in the pathogenesis of idiopathic pulmonary fibrosis. Am J Physiol Lung Cell Mol Physiol 2012;302(8):L721–9.

97. Lawson WE, Crossno PF, Polosukhin VV, et al. Endoplasmic reticulum stress in alveolar epithelial cells is prominent in IPF: association with altered surfactant protein processing and herpesvirus infection. Am J Physiol Lung Cell Mol Physiol 2008;294(6):L1119–26.

98. Kropski JA, Lawson WE, Blackwell TS. Right place, right time: the evolving role of herpesvirus infection as a "second hit" in idiopathic pulmonary fibrosis. Am J Physiol Lung Cell Mol Physiol 2012;302(5):L441–4.

99. Johnson SC, Rabinovitch PS, Kaeberlein M. mTOR is a key modulator of ageing and age-related disease. Nature 2013;493(7432):338–45.

100. Kenyon CJ. The genetics of ageing. Nature 2010;464(7288):504–12.

101. Colman RJ, Beasley TM, Kemnitz JW, et al. Caloric restriction reduces age-related and all-cause mortality in rhesus monkeys. Nat Commun 2014;5:3557.

102. Sack MN. The role of SIRT3 in mitochondrial homeostasis and cardiac adaptation to hypertrophy and aging. J Mol Cell Cardiol 2012;52(3):520–5.

103. Sack MN, Finkel T. Mitochondrial metabolism, sirtuins, and aging. Cold Spring Harb Perspect Biol 2012;4(12) [pII:a013102].

104. Rojas M, Mora AL, Kapetanaki M, et al. Aging and lung disease. Clinical impact and cellular and molecular pathways. Ann Am Thorac Soc 2015;12(12):S222–7.

105. Yoshida T, Mett I, Bhunia AK, et al. Rtp801, a suppressor of mTOR signaling, is an essential mediator of cigarette smoke-induced pulmonary injury and emphysema. Nat Med 2010;16(7):767–73.

106. Kuwano K, Araya J, Hara H, et al. Cellular senescence and autophagy in the pathogenesis of chronic obstructive pulmonary disease (COPD) and idiopathic pulmonary fibrosis (IPF). Respir Investig 2016;54(6):397–406.

107. Eijkelenboom A, Burgering BM. FOXOs: signalling integrators for homeostasis maintenance. Nat Rev Mol Cell Biol 2013;14(2):83–97.

108. Warr MR, Binnewies M, Flach J, et al. FOXO3A directs a protective autophagy program in haematopoietic stem cells. Nature 2013;494(7437):323–7.

109. Takasaka N, Araya J, Hara H, et al. Autophagy induction by SIRT6 through attenuation of insulin-like growth factor signaling is involved in the regulation of human bronchial epithelial cell senescence. J Immunol 2014;192(3):958–68.

110. Yokoyama NN, Denmon A, Uchio EM, et al. When anti-aging studies meet cancer chemoprevention: can anti-aging agent kill two birds with one blow? Curr Pharmacol Rep 2015;1(6):420–33.

111. Li S, Geng J, Xu X, et al. miR-130b-3p modulates epithelial-mesenchymal crosstalk in lung fibrosis by targeting IGF-1. PLoS One 2016;11(3):e0150418.

112. Choi JE, Lee SS, Sunde DA, et al. Insulin-like growth factor-I receptor blockade improves outcome in mouse model of lung injury. Am J Respir Crit Care Med 2009;179(3):212–9.

113. Korfhagen TR, Le Cras TD, Davidson CR, et al. Rapamycin prevents transforming growth factor-alpha-induced pulmonary fibrosis. Am J Respir Cell Mol Biol 2009;41(5):562–72.
114. Braidy N, Guillemin GJ, Mansour H, et al. Age related changes in NAD+ metabolism oxidative stress and Sirt1 activity in Wistar rats. PLoS One 2011;6(4): e19194.
115. Zhang DY, Pan Y, Zhang C, et al. Wnt/beta-catenin signaling induces the aging of mesenchymal stem cells through promoting the ROS production. Mol Cell Biochem 2013;374(1–2):13–20.
116. Zhang DY, Wang HJ, Tan YZ. Wnt/beta-catenin signaling induces the aging of mesenchymal stem cells through the DNA damage response and the p53/p21 pathway. PLoS One 2011;6(6):e21397.
117. Herbst A, Pak JW, McKenzie D, et al. Accumulation of mitochondrial DNA deletion mutations in aged muscle fibers: evidence for a causal role in muscle fiber loss. J Gerontol A Biol Sci Med Sci 2007;62(3):235–45.
118. Wallace DC. Mitochondrial DNA mutations in disease and aging. Environ Mol Mutagen 2010;51(5):440–50.
119. Panduri V, Liu G, Surapureddi S, et al. Role of mitochondrial hOGG1 and aconitase in oxidant-induced lung epithelial cell apoptosis. Free Radic Biol Med 2009; 47(6):750–9.
120. Kang MJ, Shadel GS. A mitochondrial perspective of chronic obstructive pulmonary disease pathogenesis. Tuberc Respir Dis (Seoul) 2016;79(4):207–13.
121. Hanahan D, Weinberg RA. Hallmarks of cancer: the next generation. Cell 2011; 144(5):646–74.
122. Gogvadze V, Orrenius S, Zhivotovsky B. Mitochondria in cancer cells: what is so special about them? Trends Cell Biol 2008;18(4):165–73.
123. Vendramin R, Marine JC, Leucci E. Non-coding RNAs: the dark side of nuclear-mitochondrial communication. EMBO J 2017;36(9):1123–33.
124. Akamata K, Wei J, Bhattacharyya M, et al. SIRT3 is attenuated in systemic sclerosis skin and lungs, and its pharmacologic activation mitigates organ fibrosis. Oncotarget 2016;7(43):69321–36.
125. Chilosi M, Carloni A, Rossi A, et al. Premature lung aging and cellular senescence in the pathogenesis of idiopathic pulmonary fibrosis and COPD/emphysema. Transl Res 2013;162(3):156–73.
126. Liu H, Fergusson MM, Castilho RM, et al. Augmented Wnt signaling in a mammalian model of accelerated aging. Science 2007;317(5839):803–6.
127. Shimbori C, Bellaye PS, Xia J, et al. Fibroblast growth factor-1 attenuates TGF-beta1-induced lung fibrosis. J Pathol 2016;240(2):197–210.
128. Sato A, Hirai T, Imura A, et al. Morphological mechanism of the development of pulmonary emphysema in klotho mice. Proc Natl Acad Sci U S A 2007;104(7): 2361–5.
129. Li L, Zhang M, Zhang L, et al. Klotho regulates cigarette smoke-induced autophagy: implication in pathogenesis of COPD. Lung 2017;195(3):295–301.
130. Nyunoya T, Mebratu Y, Contreras A, et al. Molecular processes that drive cigarette smoke-induced epithelial cell fate of the lung. Am J Respir Cell Mol Biol 2014;50(3):471–82.
131. Lam AP, Herazo-Maya JD, Sennello JA, et al. Wnt coreceptor Lrp5 is a driver of idiopathic pulmonary fibrosis. Am J Respir Crit Care Med 2014;190(2):185–95.
132. Franceschi C, Campisi J. Chronic inflammation (inflammaging) and its potential contribution to age-associated diseases. J Gerontol A Biol Sci Med Sci 2014; 69(Suppl 1):S4–9.

133. Xu J, Gonzalez ET, Iyer SS, et al. Use of senescence-accelerated mouse model in bleomycin-induced lung injury suggests that bone marrow-derived cells can alter the outcome of lung injury in aged mice. J Gerontol A Biol Sci Med Sci 2009;64(7):731–9.

134. Stripp BR, Reynolds SD. Maintenance and repair of the bronchiolar epithelium. Proc Am Thorac Soc 2008;5(3):328–33.

135. Rock J, Konigshoff M. Endogenous lung regeneration: potential and limitations. Am J Respir Crit Care Med 2012;186(12):1213–9.

136. Shaykhiev R, Crystal RG. Basal cell origins of smoking-induced airway epithelial disorders. Cell Cycle 2014;13(3):341–2.

137. Paschalaki KE, Starke RD, Hu Y, et al. Dysfunction of endothelial progenitor cells from smokers and chronic obstructive pulmonary disease patients due to increased DNA damage and senescence. Stem Cells 2013;31(12):2813–26.

138. Staudt MR, Buro-Auriemma LJ, Walters MS, et al. Airway basal stem/progenitor cells have diminished capacity to regenerate airway epithelium in chronic obstructive pulmonary disease. Am J Respir Crit Care Med 2014;190(8):955–8.

139. Baarsma HA, Skronska-Wasek W, Mutze K, et al. Noncanonical WNT-5A signaling impairs endogenous lung repair in COPD. J Exp Med 2017;214(1):143–63.

140. Desai TJ, Brownfield DG, Krasnow MA. Alveolar progenitor and stem cells in lung development, renewal and cancer. Nature 2014;507(7491):190–4.

141. King TE Jr, Pardo A, Selman M. Idiopathic pulmonary fibrosis. Lancet 2011;378(9807):1949–61.

142. Alder JK, Barkauskas CE, Limjunyawong N, et al. Telomere dysfunction causes alveolar stem cell failure. Proc Natl Acad Sci U S A 2015;112(16):5099–104.

143. Chambers DC, Enever D, Ilic N, et al. A phase 1b study of placenta-derived mesenchymal stromal cells in patients with idiopathic pulmonary fibrosis. Respirology 2014;19(7):1013–8.

144. Tzouvelekis A, Paspaliaris V, Koliakos G, et al. A prospective, non-randomized, no placebo-controlled, phase Ib clinical trial to study the safety of the adipose derived stromal cells-stromal vascular fraction in idiopathic pulmonary fibrosis. J Transl Med 2013;11:171.

145. Glassberg MK, Minkiewicz J, Toonkel RL, et al. Allogeneic human mesenchymal stem cells in patients with idiopathic pulmonary fibrosis via intravenous delivery (AETHER): a phase I safety clinical trial. Chest 2017;151(5):971–81.

146. Srour N, Thebaud B. Mesenchymal stromal cells in animal bleomycin pulmonary fibrosis models: a systematic review. Stem Cells Transl Med 2015;4(12):1500–10.

147. Kapetanaki MG, Mora AL, Rojas M. Influence of age on wound healing and fibrosis. J Pathol 2013;229(2):310–22.

148. Burgstaller G, Vierkotten S, Lindner M, et al. Multidimensional immunolabeling and 4D time-lapse imaging of vital ex vivo lung tissue. Am J Physiol Lung Cell Mol Physiol 2015;309(4):L323–32.

149. Yang KE, Kwon J, Rhim JH, et al. Differential expression of extracellular matrix proteins in senescent and young human fibroblasts: a comparative proteomics and microarray study. Mol Cells 2011;32(1):99–106.

150. Shapiro SD, Ingenito EP. The pathogenesis of chronic obstructive pulmonary disease: advances in the past 100 years. Am J Respir Cell Mol Biol 2005;32(5):367–72.

151. Barnes PJ. New concepts in chronic obstructive pulmonary disease. Annu Rev Med 2003;54:113–29.

152. Ramnath NW, van de Luijtgaarden KM, van der Pluijm I, et al. Extracellular matrix defects in aneurysmal Fibulin-4 mice predispose to lung emphysema. PLoS One 2014;9(9):e106054.
153. Egeblad M, Rasch MG, Weaver VM. Dynamic interplay between the collagen scaffold and tumor evolution. Curr Opin Cell Biol 2010;22(5):697–706.
154. Reticker-Flynn NE, Malta DF, Winslow MM, et al. A combinatorial extracellular matrix platform identifies cell-extracellular matrix interactions that correlate with metastasis. Nat Commun 2012;3:1122.
155. Jiang D, Liang J, Campanella GS, et al. Inhibition of pulmonary fibrosis in mice by CXCL10 requires glycosaminoglycan binding and syndecan-4. J Clin Invest 2010;120(6):2049–57.
156. Bergamaschi A, Tagliabue E, Sorlie T, et al. Extracellular matrix signature identifies breast cancer subgroups with different clinical outcome. J Pathol 2008; 214(3):357–67.
157. Sethi T, Rintoul RC, Moore SM, et al. Extracellular matrix proteins protect small cell lung cancer cells against apoptosis: a mechanism for small cell lung cancer growth and drug resistance in vivo. Nat Med 1999;5(6):662–8.
158. Parker MW, Rossi D, Peterson M, et al. Fibrotic extracellular matrix activates a profibrotic positive feedback loop. J Clin Invest 2014;124(4):1622–35.
159. Bridges RS, Kass D, Loh K, et al. Gene expression profiling of pulmonary fibrosis identifies Twist1 as an antiapoptotic molecular "rectifier" of growth factor signaling. Am J Pathol 2009;175(6):2351–61.
160. Yang J, Wheeler SE, Velikoff M, et al. Activated alveolar epithelial cells initiate fibrosis through secretion of mesenchymal proteins. Am J Pathol 2013;183(5): 1559–70.
161. Popova AP, Bozyk PD, Goldsmith AM, et al. Autocrine production of TGF-beta1 promotes myofibroblastic differentiation of neonatal lung mesenchymal stem cells. Am J Physiol Lung Cell Mol Physiol 2010;298(6):L735–43.

Epidemiology of Lung Disease in Older Persons

Carlos A. Vaz Fragoso, MD[a,b,*]

KEYWORDS

- Obstructive airway disease • Interstitial lung disease • Lung cancer

KEY POINTS

- Older persons (aged ≥65 years) have high rates of the following:
  - Respiratory risk factors: tobacco smoking, outdoor and indoor air pollution, occupational dusts, and respiratory infections.
  - Respiratory symptoms: dyspnea, chronic bronchitis, and wheezing.
  - Obstructive airway disease: chronic obstructive pulmonary disease (COPD), asthma, and the asthma-COPD overlap syndrome.
  - Interstitial lung disease: idiopathic pulmonary fibrosis, including combined pulmonary fibrosis-emphysema syndrome.
  - Lung cancer: predominantly non–small cell with advanced stages III and IV.
  - Coexisting nonrespiratory risk factors (ie, extrinsic to the lungs) that may misidentify or modify respiratory diagnoses and their clinical course: multimorbidity, polypharmacy, physical inactivity (deconditioning), reduced awareness of symptom severity, thoracic kyphosis, and frailty.

INTRODUCTION

Older persons (age ≥65 years) frequently report respiratory risk factors and symptoms and have a high prevalence of lung disease.[1–3] This article reviews the epidemiology of lung diseases that occur most commonly in older persons, including the corresponding respiratory risk factors and symptoms, as well as coexisting nonrespiratory risk factors that potentially misidentify or modify respiratory diagnoses and their clinical course.

RESPIRATORY RISK FACTORS

As shown in **Table 1**, older persons frequently report respiratory risk factors, including environmental exposures to respiratory toxins.[1,2] The respiratory system is especially

---

Disclosure Statement: No conflicts of interest.
[a] Department of Internal Medicine, Veterans Affairs Clinical Epidemiology Research Center, West Haven, CT, USA; [b] Department of Internal Medicine, Yale School of Medicine, New Haven, CT, USA
* 950 Campbell Avenue, West Haven, CT.
E-mail address: carlos.fragoso@yale.edu

Clin Geriatr Med 33 (2017) 491–501
http://dx.doi.org/10.1016/j.cger.2017.06.003
0749-0690/17/© 2017 Elsevier Inc. All rights reserved.

Table 1
Epidemiology of key respiratory risk factors for having lung disease in older persons

Respiratory Risk Factors	Comment
Tobacco smoking	• 48% to 56% are ever-smokers • 32% of non-smokers have documented exposure to ETS
Air pollution	• 80% live in metropolitan areas, a surrogate for exposure to outdoor air pollution • Among non-smokers, 18% report the use of biomass fuel for indoor cooking or heating
Occupational dusts	• Among non-smokers, 12% report a prior high-risk occupation
Infections	• 10-fold or greater rate of influenza-associated hospitalization • 27% have a history of pneumonia

Abbreviation: ETS, environmental tobacco smoke.

vulnerable to these toxins because it has the largest interface with the environment (alveolar surface area is 85 m^2 vs skin at 1.8 m^2).[4] In particular, exposure to tobacco smoke remains widespread in the current generation of older persons. In large study samples of older Americans, the prevalence of ever-smokers ranged from 48% to 56%.[1,5] Even among older never-smoking Americans, 32% had documented exposure to environmental tobacco smoke.[6] Outdoor air pollution is another common environmental exposure.[2,7] In 2014, 80% of older Americans lived in metropolitan areas, a surrogate for exposure to outdoor air pollution.[7] Additional environmental exposures include high-risk occupation (freight, stock, metal, and wood workers) and the use of biomass fuel for indoor cooking or heating.[2] The prevalence rates for these exposures in non-smoking older Americans are 12% and 18%, respectively.[2]

Respiratory risk factors also include respiratory infections, and these are highly prevalent in older persons. From the period 1979 through 2001, older Americans aged ≥75 years had a ≥10-fold increased rate of influenza-associated hospitalization, relative to any other age group.[8] In a large cohort of community-dwelling older Americans, 27% reported a prior pneumonia.[9]

In the setting of an aging lung, characterized by reduced physiologic capacity and altered immune regulation, these respiratory risk factors substantially increase the likelihood of chronic lung inflammation and the subsequent development of lung disease.[1,10]

RESPIRATORY SYMPTOMS

Dyspnea (American Thoracic Society grade 1 or higher), chronic bronchitis (cough or sputum production on most days for 3 consecutive months or more during the year), and wheezing (at any time in the past 12 months) occur frequently in older persons.[3] In a nationally representative sample of older Americans, prevalence rates were 34.2% for dyspnea, 15.1% for chronic bronchitis, and 12.4% for wheezing.[3] These respiratory symptoms are often included as diagnostic criteria in epidemiologic surveys of lung diseases, especially obstructive airway disease.[11] Importantly, epidemiologic surveys of lung diseases that are only symptom based may have limitations. For example, prior work has shown that most older persons who report dyspnea (73.0%), chronic bronchitis (67.8%), or wheezing (66.8%) have normal spirometry, yielding a positive predictive value of only 26% for any spirometric impairment (airflow obstruction or restrictive pattern).[3]

COMMON LUNG DISEASES

Table 2 summarizes lung diseases that occur commonly in older persons, including chronic obstructive pulmonary disease (COPD), asthma, asthma–chronic obstructive pulmonary disease overlap syndrome (ACOS), idiopathic pulmonary fibrosis (IPF), combined pulmonary fibrosis-emphysema syndrome (CPFES), and lung cancer.

CHRONIC OBSTRUCTIVE PULMONARY DISEASE

COPD is projected to be a leading cause of disability (fifth) and death (third) worldwide by the year 2030.[12] Older persons are at high risk of having COPD, given the age-related decline in lung function, alterations in the immune system, cumulative effects of frequent exposures to respiratory toxins, especially tobacco smoking, and high rates of respiratory infection.[1,2,5–10]

Self-Report

Epidemiologic surveys most often evaluate self-reported physician-diagnosed COPD, chronic bronchitis, or emphysema.[11] Using this approach in a nationally representative sample of older Americans, the US Behavioral Risk Factor Surveillance System estimated a prevalence of 12% for COPD in 2011.[11] It is likely, however, that a self-reported physician diagnosis of COPD is predominantly defined by clinical criteria (symptoms), given the low rates of spirometric utilization in primary care settings.[13]

Table 2
Epidemiology of common lung diseases in older persons

Lung Disease	Comment
COPD	• Self-report: prevalence of 12%[a] • Spirometry-confirmed: prevalence of 13%[b]
Asthma	• Self-report (current asthma): prevalence of 8.1%[c] • Among older persons with current asthma, the most vulnerable to adverse health outcomes are women, African Americans, Hispanics, and low-income groups
ACOS	• Among those with asthma or COPD, 17.4% have both conditions • Greater health burden, including respiratory symptoms, patient-reported outcomes, exacerbations, and comorbidities, as compared with asthma and COPD alone
IPF	• Highest annual incidence and prevalence of IPF occurs in those aged ≥75 y, ranging from 27.1 to 76.4 and from 64.7 to 227.2 per 100,000 persons, respectively
CPFES	• IPF (lower lobe fibrosis) and COPD (upper lobe emphysema) may coexist, most commonly in older male smokers • Associated with pulmonary hypertension, acute lung injury, and lung cancer
Lung cancer	• Among patients who have lung cancer, 47% are aged ≥70 y • Cancer histology (non–small > small cell) and stage distribution (predominantly stages III and IV) are comparable across age groups • Older persons are less likely to receive local therapy, despite overall outcomes for surgery or radiation being similar across age groups

[a] Of those who have self-reported, physician-diagnosed COPD, 58.6% have normal spirometry (see text).
[b] Based on spirometric z scores (see text).
[c] Of those who have self-reported current asthma, only 41.3% have spirometry-confirmed airflow obstruction (see text).

The same respiratory symptoms that potentially establish a clinical diagnosis of COPD are likely to be multifactorial in older persons, given age-related increases in multimorbidity, polypharmacy, and physical inactivity (deconditioning).[14–17] Accordingly, establishing COPD based solely on respiratory symptoms has limited diagnostic specificity in aging populations.[3] In a nationally representative sample of the US population, 58.6% of participants with self-reported, physician-diagnosed COPD had normal spirometry.[18]

Nonetheless, epidemiologic surveys of self-reported physician-diagnosed COPD should not be dismissed, because these have been shown to be clinically meaningful. In particular, self-reported physician-diagnosed COPD is associated with respiratory health care utilization and patient-reported outcomes.[19] The nuanced distinction may be that self-reported physician-diagnosed and spirometry-confirmed COPD represent separate, but overlapping, disease entities.

Spirometric Global Initiative for Chronic Obstructive Lung Disease Criteria

Because the physiologic impairment is airflow obstruction, the epidemiology of COPD has also been defined by spirometric criteria, most often using diagnostic thresholds from the Global initiative for chronic Obstructive Lung Disease (GOLD).[20] The spirometric criteria include a decreased ratio of the forced expiratory volume in 1 second (FEV_1) to forced vital capacity (FVC), defined by a GOLD threshold of less than 0.70, that is applied across all ages. COPD severity is then classified by FEV_1 percent predicted (%Pred), calculated as ([measured/predicted FEV_1] $\times$ 100%) and stratified as mild ($\geq$80 %Pred), moderate (50–79 %Pred), and severe (<50 %Pred), also applied across all ages. Using data from a nationally representative sample of Americans (Third National Health and Nutrition Examination Survey [NHANES III]), GOLD-defined COPD was established in 37.7% of older persons,[5] with most cases classified as mild COPD (49%) and only a few as severe COPD (13%).[21]

Normal aging, however, is characterized by impairments in respiratory mechanics and variability in spirometric performance.[1,22,23] The age-related impairment in respiratory mechanics includes progressive airflow limitation, manifested by a decreasing FEV_1 and FVC, as well as a decreasing FEV_1/FVC.[1] The age-related variability in spirometric performance, as measured by the coefficient of variation for FEV_1 and FVC, increases across the adult lifespan, starting at about age 40 years and occurring in all ethnic and geographically defined groups.[22,23] Hence, GOLD-based spirometric criteria lack diagnostic accuracy when establishing COPD in older persons for 2 reasons. First, the threshold of 0.70 for FEV_1/FVC fails to distinguish between age-related airflow limitation and COPD-related airflow obstruction. As a result, FEV_1/FVC less than 0.70 occurs frequently in otherwise healthy asymptomatic never-smokers, starting at ages greater than 45 to 50 years.[1,22–24] Second, because %Pred does not account for the age-related increased variability in spirometric performance, the staging of COPD severity based on FEV_1 %Pred assumes incorrectly that a given threshold value is equivalent for all persons.[1,22–25] Importantly, these age-related concerns limit the diagnostic accuracy of GOLD in establishing both the prevalence and the incidence of COPD as well as its severity, in older persons.[24]

Spirometric z Scores

To better distinguish age-related airflow-limitation from COPD-related airflow obstruction, investigators have suggested that spirometric measures be expressed as a z score, which converts a raw measurement on a test to a standardized score in units of standard deviations.[1,22,24] More recently, a method for calculating spirometric z scores was developed, termed Lambda-Mu-Sigma (LMS).[22] This strategy uses 3 elements of the distribution, including: (1) median (Mu), representing how spirometric measures change based on predictor variables (age and height); (2) coefficient of variation (Sigma), representing the spread of reference values; and (3) skewness (Lambda), representing departure from normality.[22] Clinically, z scores are already routinely used in bone mineral density testing, and the LMS method is widely applied to growth charts.[22,26]

In 2012, the Global Lung Initiative (GLI) expanded the availability of LMS-calculated spirometric z scores by publishing reference equations that included ages up to 95 years and multiple ethnic groups.[23] Using GLI equations, z scores are calculated for FEV_1, FVC, and FEV_1/FVC. The diagnostic algorithm then applies a z score threshold of -1.64, corresponding to the lower limit of normal at the fifth percentile of distribution (LLN), with airflow obstruction (COPD) defined by FEV_1/FVC z scores of less than -1.64 (<LLN).[1] COPD severity is next evaluated as a 3-level stratification, with mild defined by FEV_1 z scores ≥ -1.64, moderate defined by FEV_1 z scores less than -1.64, but ≥ -2.55, and severe defined by FEV_1 z scores less than -2.55.[27] Other FEV_1 z-score thresholds for staging COPD are available, using a 5-level severity.[28] The stated spirometric z-score thresholds have strong clinical validation, given their associations with multiple health outcomes across multiple cohorts.[1,3,5,7,17,18,27–30]

Using data from a nationally representative sample of Americans (NHANES III), z score defined COPD was established in 13.2% of older participants,[5] of whom 34% were classified as mild and 38% as severe.[29] Relative to z score defined COPD, GOLD had false positive rates for COPD of 58.4% in older Americans (NHANES III).[30]

Chest Imaging

A recent development in epidemiologic surveys has been the use of volumetric computed chest tomography (CT) to establish a diagnosis of emphysema.[27,31,32] Specifically, the diagnostic criterion is based on a calculation of percent lung having a low attenuation area of less than -950 HU ($LAA950_{insp}$), as measured on an inspiratory CT scan; percent lung values greater than 5% establish emphysema.[27,31,32] Using data from the Genetic Epidemiology of COPD study (COPDGene), which included 10,131 participants who were aged 45 to 81 years and had a smoking history averaging 44.3 pack-years, CT-diagnosed emphysema was established in 30.3%.[32]

Advancing age, however, is also characterized by structural changes in the lung, termed senile emphysema.[1] The latter relates to degeneration of elastic fibers around the alveolar duct (but in the absence of alveolar wall destruction), resulting in homogeneous airspace enlargement and reduced alveolar surface area.[1] Hence, epidemiologic surveys based on CT-diagnosed emphysema may have aging-related limitations, given that values for CT-measured $LAA950_{insp}$ may be as high as 30% in otherwise healthy persons with normal lung function.[33]

ASTHMA

Asthma imposes a substantial health burden worldwide, affecting 300 million people and ranking twenty-second in disability-adjusted life-years (similar to diabetes and Alzheimer disease).[34] In addition, 250,000 people worldwide die of asthma each year, often because of lack of treatment.[34] Regions having the highest rates of asthma include those with increased urbanization and aging populations.[34]

Self-Report

Given its high rate of urbanization and an aging population, the United States provides a unique opportunity to evaluate the epidemiology of asthma in older persons.[10] In 2014, 46.2 million Americans were aged ≥65 years, and 80% lived in metropolitan areas.[7] The United States also records detailed epidemiologic data on asthma (US National Surveillance of Asthma),[35] with the most recent decade of review covering the period from 2001 through 2010.

Using data from the US National Surveillance of Asthma and based on comparisons with other age groups, older Americans had the largest increase in the prevalence of current asthma, from 6.0% in 2001 to 8.1% in 2010.[35] Among older Americans, the highest annual prevalence of current asthma occurred in women and low-income groups.[35] Racial/ethnic differences were otherwise small (overlapping standard errors).[35]

Importantly, older Americans also had the highest rate of asthma deaths in 2009 (5.3 per 10,000 persons with current asthma), occurring more often in women and African Americans.[35] Older Americans additionally had the second highest rate of asthma hospitalization in 2009 (3.9 asthma hospitalizations as a first diagnosis per 100 persons with current asthma), occurring more often in women and African Americans.[35] Similarly, older Americans had the second highest rate of asthma-based physician office visits in 2009 (61.0 physician office visits with asthma as a first diagnosis per 100 persons with current asthma), occurring more often in women, African Americans, and Hispanics.[35]

Conversely, older Americans had the lowest rates of an asthma attack and asthma-based emergency department (ED) visits.[35] These lower rates are surprising, because they counter the noted increase in the prevalence of current asthma and the high rates of asthma-based physician office visits, hospitalization, and death in older Americans. As a potential explanation, it is postulated that older Americans had lower rates of an asthma attack and asthma-based ED visits because of an age-related reduction in the awareness of symptom severity (ie, chest tightness or discomfort, and breathlessness),[36] including as a consequence of the "paradox of well-being" (defined by high levels of life satisfaction, which may coexist with lower health expectations).[37] Because respiratory symptoms are potentially minimized in severity, the awareness of an asthma attack may be delayed in older persons, thereby decreasing utilization of ED services but subsequently increasing the rates of hospitalization and death.[10]

Spirometry

Because the predominant physiologic impairment in current asthma is airflow obstruction, the diagnostic accuracy of self-reported current asthma may be evaluated by spirometric criteria. In the Cardiovascular Health Study, which included a large sample of 4581 community-dwelling older Americans, only 41.3% of participants who had self-reported current asthma also had airflow obstruction (decreased FEV_1/FVC).[38] This low proportion may be due, in part, to participants having been evaluated during less active phases of airway inflammation (asthma is characterized by reversible airflow obstruction), or to a misdiagnosis of asthma when based solely on clinical criteria (respiratory symptoms).

ASTHMA–CHRONIC OBSTRUCTIVE PULMONARY DISEASE OVERLAP SYNDROME

Among older persons with asthma or COPD, 17.4% will have both conditions (when based on self-report), commonly referred to as ACOS.[19] ACOS may include long-standing or adult-onset asthma that has progressed to irreversible airway obstruction (vis-à-vis airway remodeling) or include COPD that is characterized by having both a smoking and an atopic history, as well as a reversible component to the airway obstruction.[39] Prior work has suggested that ACOS has a greater health burden, including respiratory symptoms, patient-reported outcomes, exacerbations, and comorbidities, relative to asthma alone and COPD alone.[19]

IDIOPATHIC PULMONARY FIBROSIS

The most common interstitial lung disease in older persons is IPF, defined as a chronic progressive fibrosing interstitial pneumonia of unknown cause.[40–42] Using a large health care claims dataset, and applying both broad and narrow case definitions, a US study estimated the annual incidence of IPF to range from 6.8 to 16.3 per 100,000 persons, whereas prevalence was estimated to range from 14.0 to 42.7 per 100,000 persons, respectively.[40] When stratified by age, however, the same study estimated the highest annual incidence and prevalence of IPF as occurring in those aged ≥75 years, ranging from 27.1 to 76.4 and from 64.7 to 227.2 per 100,000 persons, respectively.[40]

IPF also occurs more frequently in men versus women (10.7 vs 7.4 cases per 100,000 per year, respectively)[41] and in those with a history of tobacco smoking (≥20 pack-years).[42] Other putative risk factors for developing IPF include exposures to metal dusts (brass, lead, and steel), wood dust (pine), vegetable dust/animal dust, farming, raising birds, hair dressing, stone cutting/polishing, and livestock, as well as chronic viral infection, gastroesophageal acid reflux, and genetic factors (familial and sporadic cases).[42]

Given the shared risk factors of older age and tobacco smoking, IPF and COPD (in particular, emphysema) may coexist, termed CPFES.[43] This entity includes both upper-lobe emphysema and lower-lobe fibrosis and is associated with pulmonary hypertension, acute lung injury, and lung cancer.[43] It usually occurs in older male smokers.[43] The incidence and prevalence of CPFES is unknown.

LUNG CANCER

In a large US study of 316,682 patients who had a diagnosis of lung cancer, covering a 15-year period (1988–2003), age stratification showed that 45,912 (14%) were 80 years or older, 103,963 (33%) were 70 to 79 years old, and 166,807 (53%) were less than 70 years old; thus, 47% of patients with a diagnosis of lung cancer were aged 70 years or older.[44] Cancer histology (predominantly non–small cell) and stage distribution (predominantly advanced stages III and IV) were comparable across age groups, with the exception that those aged ≥80 years had a substantially higher frequency of lung cancer categorized as "not otherwise specified" (40%, as compared with 24% and 19% in those aged 70–79 and <70 years, respectively).[44]

In the same US study,[44] using an actuarial method wherein the observed survival is age adjusted for normal life expectancy, those who were aged ≥80 years had the lowest 5-year survival (7.4%, as compared with 12.3% and 15.5% in those aged 70–79 and <70 years, respectively).[44] Notably, those aged ≥80 years were less likely to receive surgical and radiation therapy (47%, as compared with 28% and 19% in those aged 70–79 and <70 years, respectively), even though 5-year survival rates were comparable across age groups for those who underwent surgery and radiation therapy, respectively.[44]

NONRESPIRATORY RISK FACTORS

Table 3 summarizes coexisting nonrespiratory risk factors (ie, extrinsic to the lungs) that may misidentify or modify respiratory diagnoses and their clinical course in older persons. Some of these factors were discussed earlier, as in multimorbidity, polypharmacy, physical inactivity (deconditioning), and reduced awareness of symptom severity.[14–17,36,37] In later discussion, thoracic kyphosis and frailty are discussed as additional age-related nonrespiratory risk factors.

The prevalence of thoracic kyphosis increases in older age, ranging from 20% to 40% and occurring as a consequence of osteoporotic vertebral deformities (especially wedging), intervertebral disk thinning, arthritis, and/or reduced muscular tone.[45–48] In a small study involving 323 older persons, wherein heart failure was an exclusion criterion, 130 (40%) had objective confirmation of thoracic kyphosis (mean age 74 years).[48] The thoracic kyphosis was associated with 230% and 130% increased odds of having spirometric airflow obstruction and restrictive pattern, respectively,

Table 3
Coexisting nonrespiratory risk factors (ie, extrinsic to the lungs) that may misidentify or modify respiratory diagnoses and their clinical course in older persons

Nonrespiratory Risk Factors	Comment
Multimorbidity	• 62% have 2 or more chronic conditions • May lead to further reductions in lung function and health status • Respiratory symptoms are likely to be multifactorial
Polypharmacy	• 20% of community-dwelling persons aged ≥65 y take 10 or more medications • 20% to 30% use medications listed in drugs-to-avoid lists • May lead to further reductions in lung function or health status • May lead to increased respiratory symptoms
Physical inactivity (deconditioning)	• Sedentary lifestyle (only 27% of Americans aged ≥75 y report regular leisure-time physical activity) • Progressive sarcopenia (frailty) • May lead to further reductions in health status • May lead to increased respiratory symptoms
Reduced awareness of symptom severity	• As in chest tightness or discomfort, and breathlessness • Paradox of well-being (high levels of life satisfaction, which may coexist with lower health expectations) • May lead to underdiagnosis or misdiagnosis of lung diseases
Thoracic kyphosis	• 20% to 40% prevalence • Associated with 230% and 130% increased odds of spirometric airflow obstruction and restrictive pattern, respectively
Frailty	• Overall prevalence of 7%, increasing more than 2-fold in those aged ≥80 y • Underlying mechanisms are likely multifactorial, but may share the final pathways of sarcopenia and osteopenia • Associated with 88% and 205% increased odds of spirometric airflow obstruction and restrictive pattern, respectively • Combined effect of frailty and spirometric impairment on mortality is multiplicative (4-fold increased risk of death)

relative to those without kyphosis.[48] In thoracic kyphosis, the airflow obstruction may be due to distortion of the airways, because these are forced to follow the abnormal curvature of the spine, whereas restrictive pattern may be due to vertebral fractures and/or decreased rib mobility.[48]

Frailty is a geriatric syndrome commonly characterized by the Fried phenotype, including the features of slow gait speed, low physical activity, exhaustion, reduced grip strength, or unintentional weight loss.[49] Based on the Fried phenotype, frailty is defined as having 3 or more of the stated features.[49] Among community living older persons, the overall prevalence of frailty is 7%, increasing more than 2-fold in those aged ≥80 years.[49] The mechanisms that underlie frailty are often multifactorial, but are likely to share the pathways of sarcopenia and osteopenia.[49] Using data from a large sample of community-living older persons, prior work has shown that frailty is associated with 88% and 205% increased odds of spirometric airflow obstruction and restrictive pattern, respectively, relative to those without any frailty feature.[7] In addition, this same study showed that the combined effect of frailty and spirometric impairment (airflow obstruction or restrictive pattern) on death was multiplicative; specifically, those who were frail and had a spirometric impairment had a nearly 4-fold increased risk of death, relative to those who had no frailty features and had normal spirometry.[7]

SUMMARY

Older persons frequently report respiratory risk factors and symptoms and have a high prevalence of lung disease, most commonly obstructive airway disease, interstitial lung disease, and lung cancer. Notably, coexisting age-related nonrespiratory risk factors are also prevalent and may misidentify or modify respiratory diagnoses and their clinical course.

REFERENCES

1. Vaz Fragoso CA, Gill T. Respiratory impairment and the aging lung: a novel paradigm for assessing pulmonary function. J Gerontol A Biol Sci Med Sci 2012;67:264–75.
2. Celli BR, Halbert RJ, Nordyke RJ, et al. Airway obstruction in never smokers: results from the third national health and nutrition examination survey. Am J Med 2005;118:1364–72.
3. Marcus BS, McAvay G, Gill TM, et al. Respiratory symptoms, spirometric respiratory impairment, and respiratory disease in middle- and older-aged persons. J Am Geriatr Soc 2015;63:251–7.
4. West JB. Respiratory physiology: the essentials. 8th edition. Baltimore (MD): Lippincott Williams and Wilkins; 2008.
5. Vaz Fragoso CA, Concato J, McAvay G, et al. The ratio of FEV_1 to FVC as a basis for establishing chronic obstructive pulmonary disease. Am J Respir Crit Care Med 2010;181:446–51.
6. Kaufmann RB, Babb S, O'Halloran A, et al. Vital signs: nonsmokers' exposure to secondhand smoke: United States, 1999-2008. MMWR Morb Mortal Wkly Rep 2010;59(35):1141–6.
7. A profile of older Americans: 2015. U.S. Department of Health and Human Services. Available at: http://www.aoa.gov/Aging_Statistics/Profile/. Accessed October 31, 2016.
8. Thompson WW, Shay DK, Weintraub E, et al. Influenza-associated hospitalizations in the United States. JAMA 2004;292:1333–40.
9. Vaz Fragoso CA, Enright P, McAvay G, et al. Frailty and respiratory impairment in older persons. Am J Med 2012;125:79–86.

10. Skloot GS, Busse PJ, Braman SS, et al. An official American Thoracic Society workshop report: evaluation and management of asthma in the elderly. Ann Am Thorac Soc 2016;13(11):2064–77.
11. Kosacz NM, Punturieri A, Croxton TL, et al. Chronic obstructive pulmonary disease among adults — United States, 2011. MMWR Morb Mortal Wkly Rep 2012;61(46):938–43.
12. Global Brief for World Health Day 2012. Geneva (Switzerland): WHO. Available at: http://www.who.int/ageing/publications/whd2012_global_brief/en/. Accessed November 1, 2016.
13. Ferguson GT, Enright PL, Buist AS, et al. Office spirometry for lung health assessment in adults: a consensus statement from the National Lung Health Education Program. Chest 2000;117:1146–61.
14. Vogeli C, Shields AE, Lee TA, et al. Multiple chronic conditions: prevalence, health consequences, and implications for quality, care management, and costs. J Gen Intern Med 2007;22(Suppl 3):391–5.
15. Steinman MA, Hanlon JT. Managing medications in clinically complex elders. JAMA 2010;304(14):1592–601.
16. Cruz-Jentoft AJ, Baeyens JP, Bauer JM, et al. Sarcopenia: European consensus on definition and diagnosis. Age Ageing 2010;39:412–23.
17. Vaz Fragoso CA, Araujo KLB, Leo-Summers L, et al. Lower extremity muscle function and dyspnea in older persons. J Am Geriatr Soc 2015;63:1628–33.
18. Vaz Fragoso CA, McAvay G, Gill TM, et al. Ethnic differences in respiratory impairment. Thorax 2014;69:55–62.
19. Vaz Fragoso CA, Murphy TE, Agogo GO, et al. Asthma-COPD overlap syndrome in the United States: a prospective population-based analysis of patient-reported outcomes and healthcare utilization. Int J Chron Obstruct Pulmon Dis 2017;12: 517–27.
20. Vogelmeier CF, Criner GJ, Martinez FJ, et al. GOLD executive summary. Global strategy for the diagnosis, management, and prevention of chronic obstructive pulmonary disease 2017 report. Am J Respir Crit Care Med 2017;195(5):557–82.
21. Ford ES, Mannino DM, Wheaton AG, et al. Trends in the prevalence of obstructive and restrictive lung function among adults in the United States. Chest 2013; 143(5):1395–406.
22. Stanojevic S, Wade A, Stocks J, et al. Reference ranges for spirometry across all ages. Am J Respir Crit Care Med 2008;177:253–60.
23. Quanjer PH, Stanojevic S, Cole TJ, et al. Multi-ethnic reference values for spirometry for the 3-95 year age range: the global lung function 2012 equations. Eur Respir J 2012;40(6):1324–43.
24. Vaz Fragoso CA. Epidemiology of chronic obstructive pulmonary disease (COPD) in aging populations. COPD 2016;13(2):125–9.
25. Miller MR, Pincock AC. Predicted values: how should we use them? Thorax 1988; 43:265–7.
26. Cummings SR, Bates D, Black DM. Clinical use of bone densitometry: scientific review. JAMA 2002;288:1889–97.
27. Vaz Fragoso CA, McAvay G, Van Ness PH, et al. Phenotype of spirometric impairment in an aging population. Am J Respir Crit Care Med 2016;193(7):727–35.
28. Quanjer PH, Pretto JJ, Brazzale DJ, et al. Grading the severity of airways obstruction: new wine in new bottles. Eur Respir J 2014;43:505–12.
29. Vaz Fragoso CA, Concato J, McAvay G, et al. Staging the severity of chronic obstructive pulmonary disease in older persons based on spirometric Z-scores. J Am Geriatr Soc 2011;59:1847–54.

30. Vaz Fragoso CA, Gill TM, McAvay G, et al. Respiratory impairment and mortality in older persons: a novel spirometric method. J Investig Med 2011;59(7): 1089–95.
31. Regan EA, Hokanson JE, Murphy JR, et al. Genetic epidemiology of COPD (COPDGene) study design. COPD 2010;7:32–43.
32. Vaz Fragoso CA, McAvay G, Van Ness PH, et al. Phenotype of normal spirometry in an aging population. Am J Respir Crit Care Med 2015;192(7):817–25.
33. Mishima M, Hirai T, Itoh H, et al. Complexity of terminal airspace geometry assessed by lung computed tomography in normal subjects and patients with chronic obstructive pulmonary disease. Proc Natl Acad Sci U S A 1999;96: 8829–34.
34. Bousquet J, Khaltaev N. Global surveillance, prevention and control of chronic respiratory diseases: a comprehensive approach. Geneva (Switzerland): WHO; 2007.
35. Moorman JE, Akinbami LJ, Bailey CM, et al. National surveillance of asthma: United States, 2001–2010. Vital Health Stat 3 2012;3(35):1–58.
36. Connolly MJ, Crowley JJ, Charan NB, et al. Reduced subjective awareness of bronchoconstriction provoked by methacholine in elderly asthmatic and normal subjects as measured on a simple awareness scale. Thorax 1992;47:410–3.
37. Levy BR. Mind matters: cognitive and physical effects of aging self stereotypes. J Gerontol B Psychol Sci Soc Sci 2003;58:203–11.
38. Enright PL, McClelland RL, Newman AB, et al. Underdiagnosis and undertreatment of asthma in the elderly. Chest 1999;116(3):603–13.
39. Postma DS, Rabe KF. The asthma–COPD overlap syndrome. N Engl J Med 2015; 373:1241–9.
40. Raghu G, Weycker D, Edelsberg J, et al. Incidence and prevalence of idiopathic pulmonary fibrosis. Am J Respir Crit Care Med 2006;174:810–6.
41. Coultas DB, Zumwalt RE, Black WC, et al. The epidemiology of interstitial lung diseases. Am J Respir Crit Care Med 1994;150:967–72.
42. Raghu G, Collard HR, Egan JJ, et al. An official ATS/ERS/JRS/ALAT statement: idiopathic pulmonary fibrosis: evidence-based guidelines for diagnosis and management. Am J Respir Crit Care Med 2011;183:788–824.
43. Jankowich MD, Rounds SIS. Combined pulmonary fibrosis and emphysema syndrome. Chest 2012;141(1):222–31.
44. Owonikoko TK, Ragin CC, Belani CP, et al. Lung cancer in elderly patients: an analysis of the surveillance, epidemiology, and end results database. J Clin Oncol 2007;25:5570–7.
45. Puche RC, Morosano M, Masoni A, et al. The natural history of kyphosis in postmenopausal women. Bone 1995;17:239–46.
46. Ismail AA, Cooper C, Felsenberg D, et al. Number and type of vertebral deformities: epidemiological characteristics and relation to back pain and height loss. Osteoporos Int 1999;9:206–13.
47. Katzman WB, Wanek L, Shepherd JA, et al. Age-related hyperkyphosis: its causes, consequences, and management. J Orthop Sports Phys Ther 2010; 40(6):352–60.
48. Di Bari M, Chiarlone M, Matteuzzi D, et al. Thoracic kyphosis and ventilatory dysfunction in unselected older persons: an epidemiological study in Dicomano, Italy. J Am Geriatr Soc 2004;52:909–15.
49. Fried L, Tangen M, Walston J, et al. Frailty in older adults: evidence for a phenotype. J Gerontol Med Sci 2001;56A:M146–56.

Evaluation of Dyspnea in the Elderly

Donald A. Mahler, MD[a,b],*

KEYWORDS

- Demand to breathe • Ability to breathe • Dyspnea domains and descriptors
- Prevalence of dyspnea • Pursed-lips breathing • Exercise training
- Inspiratory muscle training • Acupuncture

KEY POINTS

- Dyspnea is due to an imbalance between the *demand to breathe* and the *ability to breathe*.
- The 3 domains of dyspnea are sensory (intensity and qualities), affective (unpleasantness), and impact/burden with activities of daily living.
- Approximately 30% of those 65 years or older report breathing discomfort with walking on a level surface or up an incline.
- The 5 major etiologies for chronic dyspnea in the elderly include anemia, cardiovascular disease, deconditioning, psychological disorders, and respiratory diseases.
- Initial treatments to relieve breathing discomfort should be directed toward improving the pathophysiology of the underlying disease.

WHAT IS DYSPNEA?

Breathing is normally an unconscious activity. Groups of neurons in the brainstem provide automatic command that control the cyclic contraction and relaxation of the respiratory muscles. Any perturbation or dysfunction in this process can lead to the experience of breathing difficulty. Words describing discomfort associated with breathing date to circa 3300 BC, being found in the hieroglyphics of Mesopotamia. Certainly, the literal meaning, disordered (-dys) breathing (-pnea), does not capture the sensory experience of the individual. Those who experience breathing discomfort often find it hard to describe "what it feels like." Commonly used phrases are, "I am short of breath" or "I feel like I can't get enough air."

Disclosure: The author has nothing to disclose.
[a] Geisel School of Medicine at Dartmouth, 1 Rope Ferry Road, Hanover, NH 03755, USA;
[b] Department of Respiratory Services, Valley Regional Hospital, 243 Elm Street, Claremont, NH 03743, USA
* Department of Respiratory Services, Valley Regional Hospital, 243 Elm Street, Claremont, NH 03743.
E-mail address: mahlerdonald@gmail.com

In medical practice, most health care providers focus on how dyspnea affects an individual's ability to perform daily and recreational activities (impact or burden domain).

Various guidelines and strategies emphasize assessing dyspnea related to daily activities to categorize individual patients.[1–3] It is important to recognize that breathing difficulty is a strong predictor of mortality in the elderly who have no known cardiorespiratory disease,[4] in those with chronic obstructive pulmonary disease (COPD),[5] and in individuals admitted to Chest Pain Units for suspected acute coronary syndrome.[6]

In a 2012 update, the American Thoracic Society reaffirmed the following definition of dyspnea[7]:

A subjective experience of breathing discomfort that consists of qualitatively distinct sensations that vary in intensity.

It is a warning signal that the usual unconscious awareness of breathing has been altered. The update recommended that dyspnea be evaluated across 3 different domains[7]:

1. Sensory: intensity and qualities
2. Affective: unpleasantness or distress
3. Impact or burden: on activities of daily living

The objective of this article was to provide an update on the evaluation of chronic dyspnea in elderly individuals.[8–10] *Chronic* means that the symptom has been present for at least 1 month.[11] Specific topics include mechanisms of dyspnea, descriptors of breathing discomfort, unique features of dyspnea in the elderly, a diagnostic approach to assess an elderly patient with breathlessness, and treatment options to relieve dyspnea.

MECHANISMS OF DYSPNEA

A neurobiological model is often used to describe the perception of dyspnea.[12] **Fig. 1** shows a simplified model that depicts afferent impulses transmitting information from activated sensory receptors in the respiratory system to the central nervous system (CNS) and efferent impulses that travel from the CNS to the muscles of respiration. An imbalance between the *demand to breathe* and the *ability to breathe* is a plausible explanation that explains the experience of breathing discomfort. This has been called "neuromechanical dissociation."[7]

Sensory Receptors

A variety of stimuli activate different sensory receptors that transmit afferent information to the brain. The major stimuli and associated sensory receptors are listed in **Table 1**.[12] Hypoxemia and hypercapnia activate chemoreceptors, whereas multiple stimuli affect mechanoreceptors in the lung and respiratory muscles/chest wall.

Afferent Impulses

Afferent impulses from sensory receptors transmit information to brainstem respiratory centers that automatically adjust breathing to correct hypoxemia, hypercapnia, and acid-base abnormalities, and maintain appropriate mechanical status of the respiratory system. If ventilatory demand is increased (eg, physical exertion) or if a mechanical load is imposed (eg, bronchoconstriction or lung

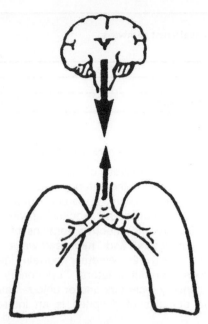

Fig. 1. Simplified model of the mechanism of dyspnea. Stimuli activate sensory receptors in the respiratory system that transmit afferent information to the CNS. After this information is processed and integrated, efferent impulses travel from the CNS to the muscles of respiration.

congestion), mechanoreceptors optimize volume and timing of breathing to minimize discomfort. Select sensory receptors and afferent pathways for transmission of impulses are listed in **Table 2**. The brainstem also can project information to higher areas in the CNS.

Table 1
Major respiratory stimuli and corresponding sensory receptors that provoke dyspnea

Stimuli	Sensory Receptors
Hypoxemia	Peripheral chemoreceptors: carotid and aortic bodies
Hypercapnia	Central chemoreceptors: medulla and midbrain
Lung inflation	Lung mechanoreceptors[a]
Airway collapse	Lung mechanoreceptors[a]
Irritant substances	Bronchial and pulmonary C-fibers
Lung congestion (eg, edema)	Pulmonary C-fibers (J receptors)
Distension of vascular structures	Pulmonary/cardiac vascular receptors
Change in muscle length (eg, hyperinflation)	Respiratory muscle spindles
Change in muscle force	Respiratory muscle tendon organs
Metabolic activity	Metaboreceptors in respiratory muscles
Emotions (eg, anger or fear)	Limbic system

[a] Includes rapidly adapting stretch receptors, slowly adapting stretch receptors, and polymodal Aδ-fibers.

Table 2
Select sensory receptors and afferent pathways

Sensory Receptors	Afferent Pathways
Peripheral chemoreceptors	Glossopharyngeal nerve
Lung mechanoreceptors	Vagal nerve
Mechanoreceptors of the diaphragm	Cervical nerves 3–5

Integration and Processing Within the Central Nervous System

Neuroimaging has shown that certain areas of the CNS are activated in response to different perturbations. These include the anterior insular cortex, amygdala, dorsolateral prefrontal cortex, and cerebellum. A cortical-limbic model has been proposed to conceptualize the integration and processing with the CNS.[13]

In addition, the discriminatory and affective domains of dyspnea appear to be processed via distinct receptors and neuropathways along with specific areas within the CNS[14,15] (**Fig. 2**). Whether certain interventions (eg, anti-inflammatory medications, bronchodilators, pulmonary rehabilitation, and opioids) act via specific sensory receptors and/or unique neuropathways to relieve sensory and/or affective domains of dyspnea is an interesting, but unproven, consideration.

Psychological Factors

Emotions can affect the perception of dyspnea, as breathing is under the behavioral control of the CNS. For example, higher levels of anxiety are associated with more intense breathlessness in those with COPD.[16,17] Anxious individuals may fear social situations because of concern that emotions may trigger or aggravate breathing discomfort. Also, unpleasantness of breathing may provoke anxiety and engender fear/panic.

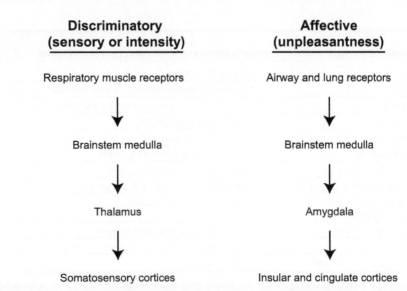

Discriminatory (sensory or intensity)

Respiratory muscle receptors
↓
Brainstem medulla
↓
Thalamus
↓
Somatosensory cortices

Affective (unpleasantness)

Airway and lung receptors
↓
Brainstem medulla
↓
Amygdala
↓
Insular and cingulate cortices

Fig. 2. Diagram of pathways for the discriminatory and affective domains of dyspnea.

Neuromodulation

Neuromodulation is the process in which different neuropeptides are secreted by groups of neurons and then diffuse across a synaptic space to produce cellular and perceptual effects. Studies have shown that endogenous opioids (naturally occurring narcotic substances) modulate the perception of dyspnea in those with COPD.[18,19] Patients reported higher ratings of breathing difficulty during treadmill exercise and while breathing through a resistance system when intravenous naloxone (an opioid antagonist) was administered compared with normal saline.[18,19] This neuromodulation appears to occur in the CNS rather than in opioid receptors in the respiratory system (bronchioles and alveolar walls).[20]

Substance P is another candidate neuropeptide for modulating dyspnea, as it augments tidal volume and respiratory frequency. Using oral aprepitant to block neurokinin-1, the receptor for substance P, there were no differences in the intensity and unpleasantness of breathlessness reported by patients with COPD compared with normal saline during resistive load breathing.[21] It is possible, although unproven, that other inhibitory and/or excitatory neuropeptides modulate the perception of dyspnea.

DESCRIPTORS OF DYSPNEA

Many individuals find it hard to describe their breathing discomfort; however, patients with different cardiorespiratory diseases are able to select statements about dyspnea that reflect their breathing experiences. The major qualities of dyspnea are summarized in **Box 1**.[22] For example, "work and effort" associated with breathing is common to various cardiorespiratory diseases. This quality reflects the important role of the respiratory muscles in the perception of breathing discomfort regardless of the underlying disease. Another feature is "chest tightness," which is unique for those with asthma.[23] A third quality is "unsatisfied inspiration," which is dominant at the end of an exercise

---

Box 1
Major qualities of dyspnea

Work/effort

1. "Work/effort" descriptors are reported by patients across the spectrum of cardiorespiratory diseases

2. This quality likely originates from respiratory muscle afferents and/or perceived cortical motor command

3. It reflects the important role of the respiratory muscles in the perception of dyspnea regardless of the underlying disease

Chest tightness

1. Typically associated with constriction of airways

2. Usually experienced in the upper anterior chest

3. Described by approximately 50% of outpatients with asthma, but not generally experienced by those with chronic obstructive pulmonary disease

Unsatisfied inspiration

1. Typically selected by patients with respiratory disease at the end of exercise

2. Appears to overlap with sensation of "air hunger" produced by increased respiratory drive such as breathing carbon dioxide

test.[24] The descriptor "air hunger" associated with breathing high levels of carbon dioxide is thought to be similar to "unsatisfied inspiration."[7]

In addition, affective descriptors, such as "frightening" (61% vs 31%, $P = .002$) and "awful" (66% vs 37%, $P = .004$) were reported more frequently in those with high anxiety scores compared with low anxiety scores.[23] Asking patients to select specific descriptors of their experience of dyspnea from a list may be helpful in the clinic to direct specific testing to establish a cause for chronic exertional breathlessness.

UNIQUE FEATURES OF DYSPNEA IN THE ELDERLY
Prevalence of Dyspnea

Estimates of the prevalence of breathing discomfort in the elderly include healthy individuals with no known cardiac or respiratory disease. The reported prevalence depends on many factors, including the definition of breathing difficulty used in questionnaires, general activity level, smoking status, occupation, geographic location, and any exposure to airborne irritants/pollutants. For populations 65 years or older, approximately 30% report breathlessness with various activities of daily living, including walking on a level surface or up an incline.[10] The prevalence of up to one-third of older people living in the community who report breathlessness with exertion is similar in residents of France, the United Kingdom, and the United States. Overall, the medical complaint of breathing discomfort is more common in women than in men.[25] It is likely that the 30% prevalence of dyspnea in the elderly is multifactorial, including possible undiagnosed cardiac or respiratory disease, decreased physical activity with low fitness levels, and increased body mass index.

Impact of Dyspnea

Breathing difficulty is 1 of the top 5 complaints among the elderly for seeking care in a general practice.[26] However, older adults ($\geq$65 years) with chronic lung disease are less likely to report that their breathing problem stops them from doing most activities compared with younger adults (<65 years).[27] Among 3600 residents who were $\geq$65 years old living in southwestern France, the risk of mortality over 13 years increased with higher levels of self-reported breathlessness.[4] This observation was independent of age, sex, body mass index, antecedent cardiovascular disease, and smoking history.[4]

Respiratory Sensation

Laboratory studies have been used to evaluate the ability of individuals to judge or rate the magnitude of added respiratory loads (breathing through different levels of resistance). In general, older individuals provide lower ratings of breathing difficulty for the same resistive load compared with younger individuals.[28] Similar findings have been noted in response to hypoxic and hypercapnic stimuli.[29,30] These findings reflect a decreased sensitivity to mechanical and chemical stimuli with advancing age.

Dyspnea During Exercise

Older healthy individuals exhibit higher levels of ventilation during exercise compared with younger subjects.[31,32] For example, the ventilatory response relative to carbon dioxide production ($\Delta\,V_E/\Delta\,VCO_2$) during exercise is substantially higher in elderly subjects ($\sim$30) compared with young subjects ($\sim$25).[31] However, older subjects report higher ratings of breathlessness for equivalent levels of power production (work/time) during cycle ergometry.[33,34] The increased respiratory demand coupled with diminished ventilatory capacity (decreases in forced vital capacity and respiratory muscle strength with aging) likely contribute to higher ratings of dyspnea during exertion.

APPROACH TO THE ELDERLY INDIVIDUAL WITH DYSPNEA

The clinical approach to the elderly individual who complains of breathing discomfort includes a medical history, physical examination, and appropriate testing. The evaluation should be directed as finding an explanation for chronic dyspnea. In particular, 5 major etiologies should be considered: anemia, cardiovascular disease, deconditioning, psychological disorders (anxiety and hyperventilation syndrome), and respiratory disease.[11] The health care provider should not assume that a complaint of breathlessness is simply due to "getting old."

The cognitive process whereby the health care provider integrates available information is based on knowledge and experience. After completion of the medical history and physical examination, the health care provider should develop a "working hypothesis" as the most likely cause of the individual's dyspnea.[10,11] Targeted diagnostic testing is recommended rather than a "shotgun" approach of ordering numerous tests to investigate for multiple possibilities.

Medical History

A comprehensive medical history is the starting point for evaluating an elderly person who complains of chronic dyspnea. First, it is important to determine whether "an awareness of breathing" is normal and appropriate. For example, someone may note breathing difficulty only with vigorous activities, such as walking up 1 or more flights of stairs, playing tennis, or hiking. The physical demands of such activities include an increase in ventilation to provide oxygen to exercising muscles. In contrast, "difficult or labored" breathing should be considered abnormal and likely due to a specific medical condition.

Next, the health care provider should ask about various characteristics of dyspnea as listed in **Box 2**.[11] The patient's responses help to clarify the impact of breathlessness on the individual's daily activities. It is helpful to ask the patient 2 questions:

- "What are your daily activities?"
- "Have you stopped doing any activities because of breathing discomfort?"

Box 2
Characteristics of dyspnea

1. Onset: When did it start?

2. Descriptor qualities: What does it feel like?

3. Frequency: How often does it occur?

4. Intensity: How bad is it?

5. Duration: How long does it last?

6. Triggers: What brings on or triggers dyspnea?

7. Associated respiratory symptoms: Do you cough? Is the cough dry or do you cough up mucus? What color is the mucus? Do you wheeze? Are you able to lie flat in bed or do you use extra pillows or support? Do you wake up in the middle of the night due to breathing discomfort?

8. Strategies that relieve dyspnea: What can you do to make it easier to breathe?

These 2 questions address the fact that individuals typically reduce or stop activities to minimize or avoid breathing difficulty. Additional information about cigarette smoking, possible inhalational exposures, occupation(s), diet, and hobbies is important. The presence of orthopnea raises the possibilities of congestive heart failure, COPD, and respiratory muscle weakness, and also can be reported in those with morbid obesity.

More than one process or cause could contribute to chronic dyspnea. Therefore, it is important to avoid *premature closure* in which a primary diagnosis is accepted before it has been confirmed.[11] Factors that help to alleviate breathlessness may enhance the medical history to identify the diagnosis.

Physical Examination

The physical examination should include the upper respiratory tract, neck, thorax, lungs, heart, abdomen, extremities, and skin. Specific abnormal physical findings are described in **Table 3**.[11] The neck examination may reveal a shift of the trachea, adenopathy, jugular venous distension, or an enlarged thyroid gland. Hypertrophy and/or active use of the sternocleidomastoid muscles, accessory muscles of respiration, are associated with severe respiratory impairment. Examination of the thorax may reveal an increase in anterior-posterior diameter that may be due hyperinflation of the lungs as well as a chest deformity, such as kyphoscoliosis.

Wheezing on auscultation indicates turbulent airflow, which may occur in asthma, COPD, and heart failure. However, the absence of wheezing does not exclude these conditions. Crackles are due to popping open of the small airways during inspiration. If they are heard throughout the inspiratory phase, consider interstitial lung disease and left-sided congestive heart failure. Crackles heard early during inspiration at the posterior bases may occur in COPD. The cardiac examination should focus on heart rhythm, point of maximal impulse, any heart murmur, and possible gallop. Clubbing of the fingers can occur in lung cancer, chronic respiratory infections like bronchiectasis and tuberculosis, interstitial lung disease, and congenital cyanotic heart disease, but not COPD. Pallor of the skin and fingernails suggests a low hemoglobin level.

In general, the lung examination is normal in those with COPD unless the forced expiratory volume in 1 second (FEV_1) is less than 50% of the predicted value.[35] In those with advanced COPD, patients may exhibit pursed-lips breathing, an increase in anterior-posterior diameter of the chest, and prolonged expiratory phase.

Suspected Anemia

Hemoglobin is a protein in red blood cells that transports oxygen throughout the body. Oxygen content is dependent on number of grams of hemoglobin, oxygen saturation, and partial pressure of oxygen. The reduced oxygen content in anemia can affect cellular function, particularly with physical tasks or exercise, because active muscles require more oxygen than is needed at rest. The body compensates for the low oxygen content by 2 major responses:

- ↑ ventilation in an attempt to inhale more oxygen into the body
- ↑ heart rate in an attempt to deliver more oxygen to the muscles

The enhanced ventilation likely contributes to shortness of breath due to an imbalance between a greater *demand to breathe* relative to the *ability to breathe*.

Major reasons to suspect anemia include recent history of bleeding and surgery in the past 3 months. A thorough dietary history along with a description of the color of the stool is important if anemia is suspected. Patients with iron deficiency frequently chew or suck on ice. With vitamin B-12 deficiency, there may be early graying of

Table 3
Abnormal physical findings observed in conditions that may cause chronic dyspnea

Findings	Condition
Mouth	
Pursed-lips breathing	Chronic obstructive pulmonary disease (COPD)
Neck	
Enlarged thyroid gland	Hyperthyroidism or hypothyroidism
Jugular venous distension	Right or left heart failure
Stridor	Upper airway narrowing
Tracheal deviation	Unilateral lung or unilateral pleural disease
Thorax	
Increased anterior-posterior diameter	Hyperinflation in COPD
Chest wall deformity	Kyphoscoliosis
Heart	
Diminished intensity of heart sounds	Hyperinflation, obesity, pericardial effusion
S_3 gallop	Ventricular dysfunction
Lungs	
Diminished intensity of breath sounds	Obesity, obstructive airway disease, restrictive ventilator defect
Prolonged expiration	Obstructive airway disease
Mid-late inspiratory crackles	Left ventricular heart failure, interstitial lung disease
Pleural rub	Pleuritis
Wheezing	Asthma, COPD, left ventricular heart failure
Abdomen	
Hepatomegaly and splenomegaly	Different causes associated with anemia
Extremities	
Clubbing	Lung cancer; chronic respiratory disease (not COPD)
Bilateral lower extremity edema	Right or left ventricular heart failure
Pallor of fingernails	Anemia
Unilateral lower extremity edema	Deep vein thrombophlebitis
Skin	
Pallor	Anemia
Petechiae	Anemia and thrombocytopenia

the hair, a burning sensation of the tongue, and loss of proprioception. Patients with folate deficiency may complain of a sore tongue and have dry scaling and fissuring of the lips. A complete blood count is required to diagnose anemia. The specific cause of anemia requires additional testing and may require a bone marrow aspiration.

Suspected Cardiovascular Disease

Risk factors for cardiovascular disease include smoking, hyperlipidemia, hypertension, diabetes, obesity, physical inactivity, being older than 55 years in women (ie, postmenopausal), and a family history of heart disease at an early age.[11] In elderly individuals, there is loss of elasticity of the myocardium and a reduced ability of the heart to respond to changes in pressure (compliance) of the arterial system. Stiffening of the arteries can lead to hypertension, which increases the work needed to pump the blood to the various organs of the body. Arteriosclerosis of the coronary arteries along with calcification of the heart valves, especially the aortic valve, are common in the elderly.

These and other processes can impair the pumping action of the heart and lead to fluid accumulation and congestion in the lungs. Fluid in the lungs activates pulmonary C-fibers (J receptors) and pulmonary/cardiac vascular receptors that cause a rapid and shallow breathing pattern. Many patients with coronary artery disease report anterior chest pain (may be described as pressure or discomfort) that typically occurs with activities and may radiate to the neck and/or the left shoulder and arm.

Suspicion of a cardiovascular etiology for chronic dyspnea should include consideration of risk factors, any report of chest pain, and pertinent physical findings.[11] Initial testing includes a chest radiograph (to estimate heart size and configuration and assessment of the pulmonary vasculature and any pleural fluid) and a 12-lead electrocardiogram (to assess for arrhythmia and ischemia). An echocardiogram is an important test to determine systolic function, chamber size, wall motion abnormalities, valve function, and an estimate of peak systolic pulmonary artery pressure. If these noninvasive tests do not establish a specific cardiovascular cause for chronic dyspnea, stress testing and/or cardiac catheterization may be required, along with consultation with a cardiologist.

Suspected Deconditioning

Deconditioning is defined as a loss of physical fitness. It is a direct result of reduced physical activities/disuse over a period of time. Deconditioning typically occurs in 2 situations: sedentary lifestyle and inactivity/rest due to acute illness, injury, or surgery. The most consistent change with deconditioning is a decline in muscle strength and mass. There is a reduced maximal oxygen uptake (Vo_{2max}) during exercise. In addition, the heart and lungs are less efficient, especially with physical exertion. With deconditioning, a higher level of ventilation is required to perform the same task compared with the previous normal fitness level.

This can cause neuromechanical dissociation between the respiratory and CNS. It is important to try to distinguish whether any loss of physical function is related to the normal decline with aging, a disease, and/or inactivity/disuse in an elderly individual. It has been estimated that approximately one-half of the decline in exercise capacity over the adult life span can be attributed to chronic physical inactivity along with the consequent increased body fat and reduced muscle mass.[36] With deconditioning, the body's metabolism slows down and weight gain is common.

Deconditioning may be suspected by asking the individual a few simple questions. Do you go for walks? Do you perform house work or yard work? Do you walk up a flight of stairs or take an elevator instead? Do you exercise at a gym or fitness center? Have you had a recent injury or illness? Did you have an operation in the past few months? Have you gained weight?

A cardiopulmonary exercise test may be useful to diagnose deconditioning.[11] Fitness can be determined by measuring the person's Vo_{2max} during incremental exercise to exhaustion. The cardiopulmonary exercise test can also provide additional information about possible cardiac or respiratory dysfunction.

Suspected Psychological Disorders

The major psychological disorders that may cause or contribute to dyspnea are anxiety and panic attacks. Anxiety disorders include generalized anxiety, panic, and social anxiety. With a generalized anxiety disorder, the individual has an abnormal and pathologic fear that interferes with the ability to function and/or to sleep. Typical feelings include worry, apprehension, irritability, and restlessness. Some elderly individuals may be overly concerned about health, money, family relations, or various social situations. Many older adults who have a chronic respiratory illness report fear of leaving home because of not being able to breathe or possibly running out of oxygen. This fear is usually magnified compared with the reality of what is happening.

In some individuals, affective responses may escalate to panic attacks that include feelings of lack of control and fear of not being able to breathe.[16] The person may have intense worries about when a panic attack will happen and may want to avoid places where panic attacks have occurred in the past. Those with social anxiety have a marked fear of social or performance situations in which the individual may expect to feel embarrassed, judged, rejected, or afraid of offending others. Anxiety and panic commonly lead to frequent hospitalizations, increased use of rescue medications, and reduced activity levels.[16]

Anxiety disorders in the elderly are frequently triggered by stress or a traumatic event such as death of a loved one, difficulties in a personal relationship, especially family members, and any medical illness, including a COPD exacerbation. The prevalence of anxiety disorders rises among older adults who have a physical illness, such as a chronic respiratory illness, particularly those in need of home health care or who live in residential care settings. For those with COPD, the prevalence of anxiety ranges from 10% to 55% depending on the patient population surveyed and the questionnaire used to diagnose the condition.[37] Anxiety is often associated with clinical depression, and studies show that depressed patients with COPD have a sevenfold risk of comorbid clinical anxiety.[38] Certainly, there is an overlap between symptoms of these 2 psychological disorders that include fatigue, weight change, sleep disturbance, agitation, irritability, and difficulty concentrating.

Physical signs of anxiety disorders reflect the body's *fight or flight* response. These include perspiration, tachycardia, and tachypnea. The rapid and shallow pattern of breathing can cause hyperinflation of the lungs in those with COPD and worsen dyspnea. Typical symptoms of anxiety are heart pounding, frequent urination or diarrhea, shortness of breath, fatigue, and trouble sleeping. Patients with COPD who report high levels of anxiety describe their shortness of breath as "My breathing is frightening" and "My breathing is awful."[23] Another common complaint is that it is "hard to get enough air in."

The diagnosis depends on the individual reporting her or his feelings to a health care provider. The health care provider may decide to test for hyperthyroidism and hypoglycemia, which can cause similar signs and symptoms associated with anxiety. Specific questionnaires are used commonly by psychologists and psychiatrists to establish a diagnosis of anxiety.

Suspected Respiratory Disease

Diseases that involve the upper and lower airways, lung parenchyma, chest wall, respiratory muscles, pulmonary vasculature, and pleural space all can cause dyspnea. As described in **Table 1**, there are many receptors in the respiratory system that may be activated to cause breathing difficulty. Major risk factors for respiratory disease are smoking, inhalational exposures, both occupational and recreational (eg, biomass fuel smoke), and a relevant family history.

A variety of pulmonary function tests are used to evaluate for suspected respiratory disease. Spirometry is usually the initial diagnostic test. An FEV_1/forced vital capacity (FVC) ratio below the lower limit of normal indicates airflow obstruction. The health care provider must then integrate available medical information to determine whether the elderly individual has asthma or COPD. Inspection of both expiratory and inspiratory flow is important to assess for an upper airway obstruction.

A reduced FVC with a normal FEV_1/FVC ratio may be due to poor effort, a restrictive ventilatory defect, and respiratory muscle weakness. In many situations, it is reasonable to measure lung volumes to diagnose whether a restrictive process is present. The single-breath diffusing capacity for carbon monoxide is used to assess gas exchange at the alveolar-capillary interface. Reduced values are observed in anemia, emphysema, interstitial lung disease, and pulmonary vascular disease. Mouth pressures assess the overall strength of the respiratory muscles. Weakness of the breathing muscles can be observed in neuromuscular disease (eg, amyotrophic lateral sclerosis and myasthenia gravis), thyroid dysfunction, connective tissue disorder, phrenic nerve injury with unilateral paralysis of 1 hemidiaphragm, and myositis.

Thoracic imaging is also important to evaluate for suspected respiratory disease. In one study, a chest radiograph along with spirometry contributed to successful diagnosis of chronic dyspnea.[39] A high-resolution computed tomography (CT) scan of the chest is the standard test for diagnosing and differentiating the different types of interstitial lung disease. A high-probability ventilation/perfusion scan is sensitive (96%) and specific (94%) for chronic thromboembolic pulmonary hypertension.[40]

Cardiopulmonary exercise testing on the treadmill or cycle ergometer can help differentiate cardiac dysfunction, pulmonary limitation, and deconditioning as a cause of chronic dyspnea.[11] Consultation with a pulmonologist may be appropriate if initial testing does not provide a specific diagnosis.

RELIEF OF DYSPNEA

Relief of breathing discomfort is a primary concern of those who experience this disabling symptom. Initial treatments to relieve breathing difficulty should be directed toward improving the pathophysiology of the specific disease. In addition, exercise training is an effective intervention for those who are deconditioned. The benefits of cardiac and pulmonary rehabilitation programs are available in major textbooks and review articles.

Approaches for relief of dyspnea are considered in the following categories: simple and inexpensive strategies, treatments for specific conditions, and acupuncture. The rationale and supporting evidence for these strategies are provided so that the health care provider can consider which intervention is appropriate for an individual patient who remains short of breath despite best available treatment of the underlying condition.[41]

Simple and Inexpensive Strategies to Relieve Dyspnea

Air movement
A breeze coming through an open window is refreshing for many individuals and may allow for easier breathing. Similarly, a fan blowing air on the face can reduce breathing discomfort. In one study, a handheld fan directed to blow air on the face reduced breathlessness in 50 patients who had advanced heart or lung disease compared with the fan directed to blow air on the leg.[42]

Release of endorphins
Endorphins are naturally occurring opioid substances that are released into the body in response to pain, stress, and breathing difficulty. Studies show that endogenous endorphins, like morphine, affect the severity of breathlessness in those with COPD.[18,19] In addition, various triggers that have been shown to release endorphins (**Box 3**).[41]

Box 3
Triggers that release endorphins

1. Alcohol

2. Caffeine

3. Chili peppers containing capsaicin

4. Dark chocolate

5. Exercise

6. Laughter

7. Listening to soothing music

8. Massage

9. Meditation and controlled breathing exercises: Tai chi, Pilates, and yoga

10. Ultraviolet light

For example, eating dark chocolate stimulates release of endorphins that then causes release of serotonin. Both endorphins and serotonin can improve mood and provide a pleasurable feeling, which may explain why some people claim to be "addicted" to eating chocolate. Exposure to ultraviolet light also releases endorphins. Whether the release of endorphins with these "triggers" provides any relief of breathing difficulty is speculative. However, individuals may wish to try 1 or more of these activities and observe whether there is any change in shortness of breath.

Body position
The leaning forward position with hands or forearms resting on the thighs or on an object like a shopping cart can make it easier to breathe.[41] This postural relief of breathing difficulty may be related to improved efficiency of the diaphragm. Many individuals report that they can walk longer with less breathlessness when their hands are supported on a shopping cart. By positioning the hands or arms so that they are supported, the shoulders are stabilized, which allows the scalene and sternocleidomastoid muscles to contribute to inhaling air into the lungs.

Listening to music
Listening to music can have relaxing effect on the brain and enables the body to slow down both heart and respiratory rates. Music also can distract from unpleasant experiences and has been shown to reduce shortness of breath during exercise.[43] Listening to music while exercising also can take away feelings that the activity is hard or boring.[44]

Pursed-lips breathing
Pursed-lips breathing involves 3 steps, as illustrated in **Fig. 3**. Puckering the lips creates pressure inside the airways that helps to prevent collapse during exhalation. Benefits include slowing down the respiratory rate, while increasing both the volume of air exhaled and oxygen desaturation.[45]

Mindful breathing
Mindfulness is an ancient Buddhist practice that means paying attention to what is happening now. Mindful breathing is an awareness of each breath so that the focus is on the present. Audio recordings are available that can provide guidance about mindfulness. As breathing becomes relaxed, the entire body can achieve a

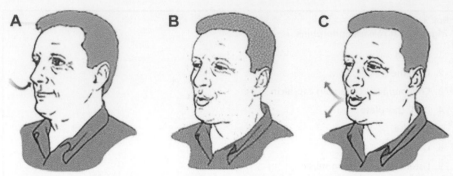

Fig. 3. Three steps of pursed-lips breathing. (*A*) Inhale through nose. (*B*) Purse or pucker lips. (*C*) Exhale through mouth.

calmness. **Box 4** describes suggestions for mindful breathing. Mindful breathing can be combined with pursed-lips breathing to ease breathing discomfort.

Relieving Dyspnea for Those With Specific Conditions

Various treatments are available to relieve dyspnea for specific conditions.

Inspiratory muscle training

Weakness of the respiratory muscles can occur with an upper respiratory tract infection, an injury to the phrenic nerve, general muscle weakness associated with deconditioning or a neuromuscular disease (eg, amyotrophic lateral sclerosis), COPD, and congestive heart failure.

Weak inspiratory muscles can cause breathing difficulty at rest, with daily activities, and/or in the supine position. Mouth pressures can be measured to assess the strength of the respiratory muscles.

Inspiratory muscle training can be performed using a handheld device. Randomized controlled trials (RCTs) have demonstrated that increasing the strength of the inspiratory muscles can improve shortness of breath. The following is a recommended training schedule: frequency, at least 5 days per week; intensity, at least 30% of maximal inspiratory muscle pressure; and duration, usually 15 minutes twice a day.[41]

Neuromuscular electrical stimulation

Some individuals, especially those with advanced heart and lung disease, may be too weak to participate in an exercise program. Neuromuscular electrical stimulation

---

Box 4
Steps for mindful breathing

1. Sit quietly in a chair or lie down.

2. Focus all attention on breathing.

3. Notice that air enters into the nose and travels into the lungs.

4. Notice that with each breath in, the stomach area moves out; and with each breath out, the stomach relaxes.

5. It is okay if your thoughts wander. Just notice the thoughts and allow them to be, and bring your awareness back to your breathing.

6. Start this exercise for a few minutes and build up each day.

provides an electrical current directly to the weak muscle via electrodes on the skin. The electrical current stimulates the muscle to contract and get stronger over time. This technique has the potential to allow those with chronic heart or lung disease who have weak muscles to increase strength, then increase physical activities, and then participate in an exercise training program. This long-term process may improve the troubling symptom of breathlessness.

Bullectomy
A bulla is an air-filled space in the lung that is at least 1 cm in diameter. **Fig. 4** shows a giant bulla that occupies approximately 30% of the right hemithorax. COPD is a common cause for a lung bulla along with alpha-1 antitrypsin deficiency (a hereditary form of emphysema), sarcoidosis, smoking cocaine, and intravenous drug use. A bulla can both compress adjacent lung tissue and cause hyperinflation of the lung, thereby shortening the length of the vertical muscles of the diaphragm. This process can contribute to shortness of breath.

Surgical resection of a large bulla (bullectomy) removes an area of nonfunctioning lung, thereby deflating the lung and enabling compressed lung to reexpand. As a result, the diaphragm muscle can lengthen and become more efficient, making it easier to breathe. The general criteria for bullectomy are a patient with the following:

- Severe shortness of breath
- A single bulla that occupies at least one-third of one side of the chest
- CT scan of the chest shows that the bulla is compressing adjacent lung

Lung volume reduction surgery
In this surgical procedure, 20% to 30% of lung tissue is resected from the upper lung zones by video-assisted thoracic surgery. The goal is to remove nonfunctioning emphysema tissue to deflate the lung so that the vertical muscle fibers of the diaphragm can lengthen and be more effective in contracting during inspiration. The National Emphysema Treatment Trial described the benefits of lung volume reduction surgery compared with continued medical therapy in 1212 individuals with severe

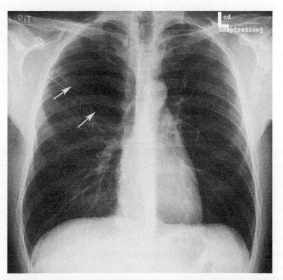

Fig. 4. A giant bulla occupies at least 30% of the right lung. Arrows indicate the lower border of the bulla in the right upper lobe.

emphysema.[46] For those individuals with emphysema mainly in the upper areas of the lung and a low exercise capacity, there were significant improvements in shortness of breath, exercise capacity, quality of life, and mortality.[46] Based on these benefits, less invasive volume reduction has been developed using placement of coils or valves into airways via a bronchoscope.

Bronchoscopic volume reduction
With bronchoscopic volume reduction, a catheter is placed through a channel of a bronchoscope to insert a one-way valve or coil into a bronchus leading to an emphysematous area of the lung. The valve or coil allows air to move out of the lung, thereby collapsing the diseased lung tissue and deflating the lung.[47] Although bronchoscopic volume reduction is widely used in Europe to treat those with advanced emphysema, at the present time, it is investigational in the United States and available only by participation in an RCT.

ACUPUNCTURE: AN EMERGING THERAPY

According to traditional Chinese medicine, *Qi* is the fundamental life energy of the universe. It is invisible and found in air, water, food, and sunlight. In the body, it is the vital force that creates and animates life. Each person is born with certain amounts of *Qi*, and it can be obtained from food and inhaled air. The level and quality of anyone's *Qi* depends on the state of physical, mental, and emotional balance. Bodily functions are regulated by *Qi* that flows from inside the body to the skin, muscles, tendons, bones, and joints by channels called *meridians*. Disruptions of this flow are believed to responsible for symptoms and disease. Dyspnea is considered to be due to a deficiency in the flow of *Qi* in the lungs.

The goal of acupuncture is to correct the imbalances in the flow of *Qi* by stimulation of locations on or under the skin. The most common technique is placement of thin metal needles that penetrate the skin. A related but different approach is to place electrode pads over the acupuncture points and then apply electrical stimulation. This is called transcutaneous electrical nerve stimulation (TENS).

There are 10 acupuncture points for the lung meridians. Stimulating these points can help to relieve breathing difficulty. To date, 6 studies have compared acupuncture or TENS over acupuncture points with a sham treatment in a total of 256 individuals with COPD.[48] In 5 of the 6 studies, there was improvement in shortness of breath with acupuncture therapy or TENS compared with the sham treatment. It is possible that acupuncture relieves shortness of breath by release of endorphins into the body, including into the cerebrospinal fluid.[49]

SUMMARY

Dyspnea is an imbalance between the *demand to breathe* and the *ability to breathe*. Approximately 30% of those 65 years or older report breathing difficulty when walking on the level or up an incline. It is likely that shortness of breath in elderly individuals is multifactorial, including possible undiagnosed cardiac or respiratory disease, decreased physical activity with low fitness levels, and increased body weight. The 5 most common causes of dyspnea in elderly individuals are anemia, cardiac disease, deconditioning, psychological disorders, and respiratory disease. Evaluation of breathing discomfort in elderly individuals includes a medical history, physical examination, and appropriate diagnostic testing.

Treatment should be directed toward improving the pathophysiology of the underlying disease. Exercise training is one of the most effective interventions, as many patients with a chronic illness are deconditioned. Simple and inexpensive strategies to relieve breathlessness include a fan blowing air on the face, pursed-lips breathing, the leaning forward position, listening to music, and mindful breathing. Inspiratory muscle training, neuromuscular electrical stimulation, bullectomy, volume reduction surgery, and acupuncture should be considered as therapies based on the individual's specific conditions.

REFERENCES

1. Vogelmeier CF, Criner GJ, Martinez FJ, et al. Global strategy for the diagnosis, management and prevention of COPD 2017 report: GOLD executive summary. Am J Respir Crit Care Med 2017;195(5):557–82.

2. O'Donnell DE, Aaron S, Bourbeau J, et al. Canadian Thoracic Society recommendations for management of chronic obstructive pulmonary disease – 2007 update. Can Respir J 2007;14(Suppl B):5B–32B.

3. Miravitlles M, Soler-Cataluna JJ, Calle M, et al. A new approach to grading and treating COPD based on clinical phenotypes: summary of the Spanish COPD guidelines (GesEPOC). Prim Care Respir J 2013;22:117–21.

4. Berraho M. Dyspnea: a strong independent factor for long-term mortality in the elderly. J Nutr Health Aging 2013;17:908–12.

5. Nishimura K, Izumi T, Tsukino M, et al. Dyspnea is a better predictor of 5-year survival airway obstruction in patients with COPD. Chest 2002;121:1434–40.

6. Hellenkamp K, Darius H, Giannitsis E, et al. The German CPU registry: dyspnea independently predicts negative short-term outcome in patients admitted to German chest pain units. Int J Cardiol 2015;181:88–95.

7. Parshall MB, Schwartzstein RM, Adams L, et al, American Thoracic Society Committee on dyspnea. An official American Thoracic Society statement: update on the mechanisms, assessment and management of dyspnea. Am J Respir Crit Care Med 2012;185:435–52.

8. Silvestri GA, Mahler DA. Evaluation of dyspnea in the elderly patient. Clin Chest Med 1993;14:393–404.

9. Mahler DA, Fierro-Carrion G, Baird JC. Evaluation of dyspnea in the elderly. Clin Geriatr Med 2003;19:19–33.

10. Mahler DA, Baird JC. Dyspnea in the elderly. In: Mahler DA, O'Donnell DE, editors. Dyspnea: mechanisms, measurement, and management. 2nd edition. Boca Raton (FL): Taylor & Francis; 2005. p. 19–28.

11. Gifford AH, Mahler DA. Chronic dyspnea. In: Mahler DA, O'Donnell DE, editors. Dyspnea: mechanisms, measurement, and management. 3rd edition. Boca Raton (FL): CRC Press; 2014. p. 145–60.

12. Mahler DA, O'Donnell DE. Neurobiology of dyspnea: an overview. In: Mahler DA, O'Donnell DE, editors. Dyspnea: mechanisms, measurement, and management. 3rd edition. Boca Raton (FL): CRC Press; 2014. p. 3–10.

13. Evans KC, Banzett RB. Neuroimaging of dyspnea. In: Mahler DA, O'Donnell DE, editors. Dyspnea: mechanisms, measurement, and management. 3rd edition. Boca Raton (FL): CRC Press; 2014. p. 11–24.

14. Davenport PW, Vovk A. Cortical and subcortical central neural pathways in respiratory sensation. Respir Physiol Neurobiol 2009;167:72–86.

15. Von Leupoldt A, Dahme B. Cortical substrates for the perception of dyspnea. Chest 2005;128:345–54.

16. Von Leupoldt A, Van den Bergh O, Davenport PW. Anxiety, depression and panic. In: Mahler DA, O'Donnell DE, editors. Dyspnea: mechanisms, measurement, and management. 3rd edition. Boca Raton (FL): CRC Press; 2014. p. 129–44.

17. Von Leupoldt A, Dahme B. Psychological aspects in the perception of dyspnea in obstructive pulmonary diseases. Respir Med 2007;101:411–22.

18. Mahler DA, Murray JA, Waterman LA, et al. Endogenous opioids modify dyspnoea during treadmill exercise in patients with COPD. Eur Respir J 2009;33: 771–7.

19. Gifford AH, Mahler DA, Waterman LA, et al. Neuromodulatory effect of endogenous opioids on the intensity and unpleasantness of breathlessness during resistive load breathing in COPD. COPD 2011;8:160–6.

20. Mahler DA, Gifford AH, Waterman LA, et al. Effect of increased blood levels of ß-endorphin on perception of breathlessness. Chest 2013;143:1378–85.

21. Mahler DA, Gifford AH, Gilani A, et al. Antagonism of substance P and perception of breathlessness in patients with chronic obstructive pulmonary disease. Respir Physiol Neurobiol 2014;196:1–7.

22. Parshall MB, Schwartzstein RM. Domains of dyspnea measurement. In: Mahler DA, O'Donnell DE, editors. Dyspnea: mechanisms, measurement, and management. 3rd edition. Boca Raton (FL): CRC Press; 2014. p. 85–98.

23. Chang AS, Munson J, Gifford AH, et al. Prospective use of descriptors of dyspnea to diagnose common respiratory diseases. Chest 2015;148:895–902.

24. O'Donnell DE, Bertley JC, Chau LK, et al. Qualitative aspects of exertional breathlessness in chronic airflow limitation: pathophysiologic mechanisms. Am J Respir Crit Care Med 1997;144:109–15.

25. Watson L, Vestbo J, Postma D, et al. Gender differences in the management and experiences of chronic obstructive pulmonary disease. Respir Med 2004;98: 1207–13.

26. Frese T, Mahlmeister J, Deutsch T, et al. Reasons for elderly patients' GP visits: results of a cross-sectional study. Clin Interv Aging 2016;11:127–32.

27. Berry CE, Han MK, Thompson B, et al. Older adults with chronic lung disease report less limitation compared with younger adults with similar lung function impairment. Ann Am Thorac Soc 2015;12:21–6.

28. Tack M, Altose MD, Cherniack NS. Effects of aging on perception of resistive ventilatory loads. Am Rev Respir Dis 1982;126:463–7.

29. Kronenberg RS, Drage CW. Attenuation of the ventilatory and heart rate responses to hypoxia and hypercapnia with aging in normal men. J Clin Invest 1973;52:1812–9.

30. Peterson DD, Pack AI, Sialge DA, et al. Effects of aging on ventilatory and occlusion pressure responses to hypoxia and hypercapnia. Am Rev Respir Dis 1981; 124:387–91.

31. Brischetto MJ, Millman RP, Peterson DD, et al. Effect of aging on ventilatory response to exercise and CO_2. J Appl Physiol Respir Environ Exerc Physiol 1984;56:1143–50.

32. Faisal A, Webb KA, Guenette JA, et al. Effect of age-related ventilator inefficiency on respiratory sensation during exercise. Respir Physiol Neurobiol 2015;205: 129–39.

33. Mahler DA, Mejia-Alfaro R, Ward J, et al. Continuous measurement of breathlessness during exercise: validity, reliability, and responsiveness. J Appl Physiol (1985) 2001;90:2188–96.

34. Fierro-Carrion G, Mahler DA, Ward J, et al. Comparison of continuous and discrete measurements of dyspnea during exercise in patients with COPD and normal. Chest 2004;125:77–84.
35. Stubbing DG, Mathur PN, Roberts RS, et al. Some physical signs in patients with chronic airflow obstruction. Am Rev Respir Dis 1982;125:549–52.
36. Gerlach Y, Williams MT, Coates AM. Weighing up the evidence—a systematic review of measures used for the sensation of breathlessness in obesity. Int J Obes 2013;37:341–9.
37. Willgoss TG, Yohannes AM. Anxiety disorders in patients with COPD: a systematic review. Respir Care 2013;58:858–66.
38. Lacasse Y, Rousseau L, Maltais F. Prevalence of depressive symptoms and depression in patients with severe oxygen-dependent chronic obstructive pulmonary disease. J Cardiopulm Rehabil 2001;21:80–6.
39. Pratter MR, Curley FJ, Dubois J, et al. Cause and evaluation of chronic dyspnea in a pulmonary disease clinic. Arch Intern Med 1989;149:2277–82.
40. Worsley DE, Palevsky HI, Alavi A. Ventilation-perfusion lung scanning in the evaluation of pulmonary hypertension. J Nucl Med 1994;35:793–6.
41. Mahler DA. Other treatments for dyspnea. In: Mahler DA, O'Donnell DE, editors. Dyspnea: mechanisms, measurement, and management. 3rd edition. Boca Raton (FL): CRC Press; 2014. p. 207–21.
42. Galbraith S, Fagan P, Perkins P, et al. Does the use of handheld fan improve chronic dyspnea? A randomized, controlled, crossover trial. J Pain Symptom Manage 2010;39:831–8.
43. Bauldoff GS, Hoffman LA, Zullo TG, et al. Exercise maintenance following pulmonary rehabilitation: effect of distractive stimuli. Chest 2002;122:948–54.
44. Singh VP, Rao V, Prem V, et al. Comparison of the effectiveness of the music and progressive muscle relaxation for anxiety in COPD—a controlled pilot study. Chron Respir Dis 2009;6:209–16.
45. Tiep BL, Burns M, Kao D, et al. Pursed lips breathing training using ear oximetry. Chest 1989;90:218–21.
46. Fishman A, Martinez F, Naunheim K, et al. A randomized trial comparing lung-volume reduction surgery with medical therapy for severe emphysema. N Engl J Med 2003;348:2059–73.
47. Deslee G, Mal H, Dutau H, et al. Lung volume reduction coil treatment vs usual care in patients with severe emphysema: the REVOLENS randomized clinical trial. JAMA 2016;315:175–84.
48. Mahler DA. A perspective on acupuncture techniques for relief of dyspnea in chronic obstructive pulmonary disease. Med Acupunct 2016;28:28–32.
49. Clement-Jones V, McLoughlin L, Tomlin S, et al. Increased beta-endorphin but not metenkephalin levels in human cerebrospinal fluid after acupuncture for recurrent pain. Lancet 1980;2:946–9.

Asthma in the Elderly

 CrossMark

Sidney S. Braman, MD, FCCP

KEYWORDS

• Aging • Asthma • Lung function • Overlap syndrome • Phenotypes

KEY POINTS

- New-onset asthma may occur at any age.
- Elderly patients with long-standing asthma usually have a history of atopy; IgE levels are elevated and often there is a history of allergic rhinitis.
- Asthma that begins at an advanced age is usually nonatopic and has low rates of remission.
- There are no specific protocols for the treatment of asthma in the elderly; treatment entails objective monitoring, avoidance of asthma triggers, pharmacotherapy, and patient education.
- Most elderly asthmatics tolerate asthma medications well with minimal adverse drug reactions.

INTRODUCTION

Asthma was long considered a childhood disease. There was little focus on asthma in elderly subjects until the Tucson epidemiologic study of obstructive lung disease brought attention to asthmatics in this age group.[1] This longitudinal study began in 1971 and results of the eighth survey in 1984 showed that active asthma is relatively common in people over age 65 years of age. Many subjects had severe disease with marked ventilatory impairment and suffered with this disabling disorder for years. Fewer than 1 of 5 in the study group went into complete remission and the death rates in the asthmatics tended to be higher than in nonasthmatics.[2] A further report of patients who developed asthma after the age of 60 showed that the serum IgE level was closely related to the likelihood of a subsequent asthma diagnosis and that a rapid decrease in lung function often occurred around the time of the initial diagnosis.[3]

The Tucson epidemiologic study offered the first characterization of asthma in the elderly (AIE) and highlighted the need for further investigation in the group. In the decades that followed, it became apparent that AIE is underdiagnosed and undertreated and that there is a paucity of knowledge regarding many aspects of the disease in this

No Disclosures.
Division of Pulmonary, Critical Care and Sleep Medicine, Department of Medicine, Icahn School of Medicine at Mount Sinai, One Gustave L. Levy Place, Box #1232, New York, NY 10029, USA
E-mail address: sidney.braman@mssm.edu

age group.[4–11] The need for an assessment of current knowledge became apparent. This resulted in a workshop convened by the National Institute on Aging in September 2008, to improve the understanding and care of AIE, defined as asthma in those over 65 years of age.[12] At that time, it was acknowledged that at least 2 phenotypes exist among elderly asthmatics, namely, those with long-standing asthma have more severe airflow limitation and less complete reversibility than those with late-onset asthma that often, as was seen in the Tucson study, can occur for the first time at an advanced age.[1,13] This raised questions regarding the pathophysiological mechanisms of AIE. Are they different from those seen in young asthmatics? And are aging-related changes in respiratory and immune physiology affecting the manifestations of this disease in the elderly?

It was acknowledged at the National Institute on Aging workshop that asthma presenting at an advanced age often has similar clinical and physiologic consequences as seen with younger individuals, but there are a number of confounding influences that complicate asthma in this age group, including the presence of comorbid illnesses. In addition, the clinical presentation may be highly variable as a result of the heterogeneity among older people that ranges from very "fit" to very "frail." In May 2015, an American Thoracic Society Workshop on Asthma in the Elderly was convened to review the current state-of-the-art knowledge and provide future directions for research.[14]

EPIDEMIOLOGY

The most recent revised global estimate of asthma from the World Health Organization suggests that as many as 334 million people have asthma, and that the burden of disability is high.[15] Asthma is especially seen with increased urbanization and with aging populations. A cohort of asthmatics in Norway followed for 11 years showed a higher risk for older patients. The incidence of asthma per 1000 person years was 2.4, 3.1, and 5.4 for age groups 15 to 29, 30 to 45, and 50 to 70 years respectively.[16] Similar estimates from the United States, Poland, and Sweden have been reported.[16] The incidence of this disease has increased substantially in recent decades.[16,17] About 250,000 asthmatics die from this disease each year, often as a result of poor access to care, poor environmental control, and a lack of proper medications.[18]

A comprehensive epidemiologic study from the United States National Surveillance of Asthma was conducted for several decades and has been reviewed in the American Thoracic Society workshop document.[17] The data on Americans across the lifespan, including those age 65 years of age and older, showed that older Americans had (1) the greatest increase in the prevalence of current asthma, from 6.0% in 2001 to 8.1% in 2010, (2) the highest rate of asthma-related deaths, and (3) the second highest rate of asthma-based physician office visits and hospitalizations, but (4) the lowest rate of having an asthma attack and an asthma-based emergency department visit, respectively. The most vulnerable of the older Americans were females, African Americans, Hispanics, and low-income groups.

In an analysis of a large US database of emergency department visits and hospitalizations for asthma between 2006 and 2008, Tsai and colleagues[19] found that patients over age 65 with asthma had higher rates and greater durations of hospitalization, greater mortality, and more near-fatal attacks.

The presence of age-associated comorbidities of AIE such as heart disease, chronic obstructive pulmonary disease (COPD), kyphosis, gastroesophageal reflux, and pulmonary vascular disease makes determining asthma-related health care use difficult. In addition, many common geriatric conditions such as cognitive impairment, falls, low body mass index, dizziness, and vision impairment can have a significant effect on activities of daily living and these conditions can be as prevalent as common chronic diseases in the elderly.[20]

PATHOPHYSIOLOGY

Asthma is caused by a complex interaction of cells, mediators, and cytokines that result in airway inflammation.[21,22] Inflammatory cells such as mast cells, eosinophils, activated T lymphocytes, and neutrophils can be seen on bronchial biopsies of asthmatic patients. Their release of specific cytokines seems to direct the movement of cells to the site of airway inflammation. Inflammatory cytokines also activate cells, causing them to further release their mediators. Mast cells, usually as a result of IgE-mediated stimulation, release preformed mediators, such as histamine, leukotrienes, prostaglandins, and proteases that promote bronchoconstriction, airway edema, mucus hypersecretion, and vascular congestion in the airways. Eosinophil infiltration is prominent in most asthmatics. Denudation of the airway epithelium can occur in severe asthma. This process can lead to airway edema and loss of substances in the mucosa that protect the airway. Epithelial damage promotes bronchial hyperresponsiveness (bronchoconstrictive responses). Increased access to sensory nerve endings may contribute to this phenomenon. Another characteristic finding in severe asthma is the presence of tenacious mucus plugs in the airways. Death from asthma usually occurs from blockage of the airways by diffuse mucus plugging. Thickening of the reticular basement membrane, the laminar reticularis, is observed on light microscopy and is a constant feature of asthma. There is also evidence of increased bronchial smooth muscle mass (hypertrophy and hyperplasia) that contributes considerably to the thickness of the airway wall. The airway architecture is also changed by the deposition of types I, III, and V collagen and fibronectin beneath the basement membrane. This has been referred to as "subepithelial fibrosis." These architectural changes collectively seen in the airways of many elderly (and some younger) asthmatics are referred to as airway remodeling and are thought to cause permanent changes that result in fixed airflow obstruction. The degree of remodeling seems to worsen with more severe degrees of asthma, although not all patients have similar changes in each component of the remodeled airway.[22]

Sputum, bronchoalveolar lavage, and bronchial mucosal biopsy specimens from elderly stable asthmatics have confirmed the presence of prominent eosinophilia, and CD4$^+$ T lymphocytes, as seen with younger asthmatics.[23] Pathologic findings have been compared in young and older subjects who have died from fatal attacks of asthma.[24] Both old and young patients with asthma have thickened airway smooth muscle compared with normal subjects. Some studies have shown that older asthmatics with a longer duration of disease demonstrate increase in airway wall thickness. Another contributing factor to fixed airflow obstruction is a loss of elastic recoil. It has been reported in chronic asthma and it may be seen in varying age groups.[25,26]

There is evidence that the airway function of young and middle age asthmatics may decline at a greater rate than normal subjects.[27–29] The rate of decline increases with increasing age and in those who smoke cigarettes.[28,30] These changes in asthmatics are variable because not all individuals show a steep rate of decline. The precise reasons for this individual variability have not been defined, although a history of atopy and marked bronchial hyperresponsiveness are 2 important risk factors for airflow obstruction.[31] The long duration and severity of previous disease are also significant factors,[32] although some elderly asthmatics with severe airflow obstruction report having had a relatively short duration of symptoms, on the order of months to a few years. In asthmatics who develop asthma later in life, there is also evidence that lung function is reduced in some even before a diagnosis is made, declines rapidly shortly after diagnosis, and thereafter remains fairly stable.[2] In general, however, those with long-standing asthma have been shown to have more severe fixed airway obstruction.[13] Airflow obstruction seen in the older asthmatic may not be attributable to asthma alone. The pathologic changes of asthma may synergize with those of normal aging, such as loss of lung elastic recoil, to affect both lung structure and function. The concept that aging and/or asthma duration can result in airway remodeling and cause "fixed" or irreversible airflow obstruction in this population can explain the lung function abnormalities seen in many older asthmatics. In a random survey of 1200 elderly asthmatics over aged 65 years from the Mayo Clinic, only 1 in 5 patients had normal pulmonary function even after administration of an inhaled short-acting bronchodilator.[33]

CLINICAL FEATURES

The typical symptoms of asthma, namely, episodic wheezing, shortness of breath, and chest tightness, are the same in older asthmatics as in younger patients.[34] Often, the symptoms are worse at night and may be precipitated by exertion. However, compared with younger asthmatics, elderly asthmatics have greater morbidity[11] and lower scores on subjective assessments of health-related quality of life.[35] In addition to asthma symptoms, the elderly asthmatic is more likely to report poor general health, symptoms of depression, and limitation of activities of daily living.[4]

The symptoms of asthma in older adults are nonspecific, however, and are common to other conditions that are frequently seen with other comorbidities common in older adults. Dyspnea, for example, is a frequent complaint in those with heart disease, and paroxysmal nocturnal dyspnea can be due to both asthma and congestive heart failure. Many older patients limit their activity to avoid dyspnea; others may assume that their dyspnea is a result of aging and avoid seeking medical attention early in their disease course. Aging, per se, does not cause dyspnea. Cough is a prominent symptom and occasionally may be the only presenting symptom.[36] Wheezing, in contrast, may not be as prominent, and its presence is not specific and does not correlate with severity of obstruction.

Asthma is often triggered by environmental exposures. The Cardiovascular Health Study general population sample of asthmatics found that asthmalike symptoms were often brought on or made worse by exposure to the following factors: dust, smoke or fumes, and contact with animals, plants, or pollens.[4] Also, similar to younger asthmatics, upper respiratory tract infections are common triggers of asthma symptoms and 1 community study showed that the majority of elderly patients who develop asthma after age 65 have their first asthma symptom preceded immediately by, or concomitant with, an upper respiratory tract infection.[6]

A history of atopy is a strong predictor of asthma in this age group, and current or previous allergic rhinitis, sinusitis, and nasal polyps are not uncommon. A comprehensive review of medications taken by patients may be helpful because aspirin, nonsteroidal antiinflammatory agents, and beta-blockers also can trigger symptoms. The physical examination in older patients who have asthma is usually nonspecific and a normal examination may obscure the diagnosis.

Studies have repeatedly shown that symptoms caused by asthma are frequently ignored or dismissed by older patients. Also, elderly patients, when compared with younger patients, have been shown to have a reduced perception of bronchoconstriction.[37] This is true in both normal subjects and in asthmatics. This can delay medical intervention. Many older patients are fearful of having an illness and dying and are reluctant to admit that they have symptoms. Even when they do so, they may underestimate the symptoms, consider them a result of normal aging, or confuse these symptoms with those of other comorbid illnesses if present. Underreporting of symptoms in older adults may have many causes, including fear, depression, cognitive impairment, social isolation, denial, and poor medical literacy.

AIE may also be overlooked or misdiagnosed by physicians. Asthma symptoms are common to other conditions seen in older patients and asthma may be mimicked by these other diseases. Conditions such as congestive heart failure, emphysema and chronic bronchitis (COPD), chronic aspiration, gastroesophageal reflux disease (GERD), and endobronchial tumors can mimic asthma. Early morning wheezing is a prominent symptom of congestive heart failure. Asthma has not been found to be a risk factor for cardiovascular disease, unless there is a smoking history or a concomitant diagnosis of COPD.[38] Typical symptoms of GERD, such as vomiting and heartburn, may be absent in older adults. Reports of older patients with esophageal reflux proven by intraesophageal pH monitoring showed that chronic cough, hoarseness, and wheezing were present in the majority of patients studied.[39,40] The relationship between GERD and asthma has been controversial. Attempts to control GERD with proton pump inhibitors (PPIs) has a limited impact on symptoms and lung function in patients with asthma and symptomatic GERD.[41]

OBJECTIVE MEASURES OF ASTHMA
Lung Function Testing

Objective measures of lung function with spirometry and peak flow measurements have been used to confirm the presence of asthma and monitor the disease. Airflow obstruction is usually present in symptomatic patients and reversibility can be shown after inhalation of a short-acting beta-agonist or anticholinergic agent. If complete reversibility of the airflow obstruction is seen, a diagnosis of asthma is more certain. COPD patients will also show airflow obstruction, but complete reversibility in not seen. Airflow obstruction is demonstrated by a reduction of the forced expiratory volume exhaled in 1 second (FEV_1) and the ratio of FEV_1/forced vital capacity (FVC). The Global Initiative for Chronic Obstructive Lung Disease (GOLD) COPD Guidelines use a fixed ratio of FEV_1/FVC of less than 70% to determine airflow obstruction.[42] However, as aging occurs there is a loss of lung elastic recoil that reduces the FEV_1/FVC ratio in normal subjects. As a result, the diagnosis of airflow obstruction can be overestimated markedly. For example, in 1 study of patients over age 80, using the fixed ratio Turkeshi and colleagues[43] found that 27% of the subjects had airflow obstruction. It has been recommended that it is best to define airflow obstruction by the lowest 5% of the reference population (the lower limit of normal).[44,45] Using this criterion to reevaluate the data, Turkeshi and colleagues[43] found airflow obstruction in only 9% of patients.

International standards regarding performance of spirometry have been published[46,47] and widely accepted. Unfortunately, spirometry is underused in older patients.[6] This contributes to the delay or failure to make a diagnosis. Although the effort-dependent maneuvers of spirometry may be difficult to perform in some patients because of physical and cognitive impairment, in 1 study a total of 585 elderly patients (81.8%) were able to perform spirometry according to accepted criteria.[48] Overall, geriatric patients are able to perform an imperfect, often unfinished, but acceptable forced expiration on this testing.[49] If airflow obstruction is found, attempts to demonstrate reversibility (postbronchodilator FEV_1 or FVC increases of >12% and 200 mL) should be made.[50] Although reversibility testing becomes increasingly difficult with age, reliable data were found in a vast majority (94%) of subjects in 1 community study.[51] A positive bronchodilator response makes a diagnosis of asthma is more secure; a negative response does not rule out asthma.[11] Unlike younger asthmatics, most elderly asthmatics show incomplete reversibility.[12] This can lead to a misdiagnosis of COPD.

Peak expiratory flow variability may be helpful in the diagnosis and follow-up of younger patients with asthma, but poor coordination and muscle weakness in some patients may lead to an inaccurate reading.[52,53] A prospective study failed to demonstrate any advantage of peak flow monitoring over symptom monitoring as an asthma management strategy for older adults with moderate to severe asthma.[54]

Airway obstruction may be absent at the time of testing and further evaluation may be needed to facilitate the diagnosis. Bronchoprovocation testing with a methacholine challenge can be useful and it is a safe, effective method to uncover asthma in older adults.[55,56] A negative test rules out asthma; a positive test must be interpreted and include an assessment of pretest probability.[57]

Use of Biomarkers

There are no particular biomarkers that distinguish younger and elderly asthmatics. AIE may be more neutrophilic,[58] but sputum neutrophil predominance is not specific to elderly asthmatics and can be found in older subjects without asthma as well,[59] and in younger asthmatics with severe disease.[60]

Blood and sputum eosinophilia are common but not universal in asthmatics at any age. Older asthmatic subjects with evidence of atopy continue to exhibit sputum eosinophil numbers comparable to those seen in younger asthmatic subjects.[61]

In a study comparing older patients (>65 years) with fixed airflow obstruction and either nonsmoking asthmatics or COPD patients, those with asthma had significantly increased blood and sputum eosinophil counts and eosinophilic cationic protein levels.[62] It seems, however, that aged eosinophils might have altered effector functions.[63] In a study examining age-related changes in eosinophil function, it was found that peripheral eosinophils from asthmatic subjects (age range, 55–80 years) exhibited decreased degranulation in response to chemotactic stimulation with IL-5 and lower superoxide production.[61] Thus, eosinophils might be less functional in the elderly but continue to be associated with asthma.

Exhaled nitric oxide (FeNO) is used as an asthma biomarker in younger patients with asthma. FeNO is most accurately classified as a marker of T-helper cell type 2–mediated airway inflammation with a high positive and negative predictive value for identifying corticosteroid-responsive airway inflammation.[64] Higher levels have been found in very elderly asthmatics (over the age of 80 years), compared with a younger cohort of asthmatics (ages 18–30 years).[65] However, Columbo and colleagues[66] found that FeNO levels did not relate to disease activity measured by symptoms, lung function or exacerbations in a year-long study of 30 stable asthmatics ages 60 years and older. A Cochrane Database review concluded that the universal use of FeNO to help guide therapy in adults with asthma cannot be advocated. The main benefit of monitoring FeNO shown in this review was to help reduce exacerbations in a subgroup of patients who suffer from frequent exacerbations.[67] Overall, studies have suggested that FeNO likely has similar monitoring capabilities in both older and younger patients with asthma.

ASTHMA PHENOTYPES

There is increasing appreciation of the heterogeneity of asthma.[68] There are many phenotypic expressions of the disease that are defined by differences in clinical presentations but give no insight into pathophysiologic mechanisms. A disease endotype is its functional or pathophysiologic mechanism. An appreciation of different disease endotypes among asthmatics has explained the differences in individual responses to various treatments and has also led to successful therapeutic trials of new biologic treatments. An appreciation of asthma phenotypes and endotypes in AIE has offered insights into the management of these patients.

Early-Onset Versus Late-Onset Asthma

The incidence of new-onset asthma is greatest in childhood and adolescence and, for many, asthma will persist into late adulthood. However asthma may develop at any age. When asthma occurs for the first time at an advanced age (>65 years) it has been labeled "late-onset asthma" and has been contrasted with "early-onset asthma" that often has been present for many decades and is more likely to have an atopic phenotype.[12,13,69] Although these groups are indistinguishable by symptoms and medication requirements, the early-onset asthmatics are more likely to have more fixed airflow obstruction on spirometry[13] and are more at risk for an acute exacerbation.[70]

Atopic Asthma

The presence of atopy is common with asthma; more than 80% of children are allergen sensitized and this has proven to be a marker of more severe disease.[71] A French study of asthma found only 14.7% of asthmatics over age 65 were sensitized to at least 1 antigen compared with 60.1% under age 21 years. Although there is a decreasing prevalence of atopy with age,[72–74] a number of studies have confirmed allergic sensitization in certain populations of elderly asthmatics. An inner-city study by Rogers and colleagues[75] demonstrated that 60% of asthmatics greater than 65 years were sensitized to at least one antigen, the most common being cockroach.

Another by Busse and colleagues[76] showed that 41% of patients with moderate to severe asthma over the age of 60 were atopic, compared with 73% of patients between ages 18 and 35. Although most elderly asthmatics develop atopy at an earlier age, it has been documented that atopy can develop later in life. In the VA Normative Aging Study of older men (mean age, 61.2 ± 8.1 years), those with newly developed airway hyperresponsiveness were more likely to have developed sensitization to cats (23.9% vs 4.4%) compared with matched controls.[77]

Obesity and Asthma

Obesity is a major risk factor for asthma.[78] The phenotypic features of the obese asthmatic are late-onset nonatopic asthma that is poorly controlled and often corticosteroid dependent. There is a predominance of female patients and often quality of life is poor and health care use high. Although obesity is known to adversely affect lung mechanics, it is also known to be a proinflammatory state.

The fact that weight reduction improves asthma control suggests involvement of inflammatory pathways secondary to obesity in the pathogenesis of asthma.[79] A Korean Longitudinal Study on Health and Aging (age >65 years) showed that the risk of asthma increased in proportion to the increase in body mass index in this elderly population. Additional studies specific to this age group are needed. Another phenotype of obesity and AIE occurs when a severe corticosteroid-dependent asthmatic remains on the corticosteroids for years and gains excessive weight as a complication of this treatment. There has been little research directed toward this problem.

Aspirin-Exacerbated Respiratory Disease

The association of aspirin and asthma was made by Samter and Beers in 1968 and was formerly called Samter triad.[80] The features of this syndrome include severe chronic rhinosinusitis and nasal polyposis, asthma and an exacerbation of severe asthma symptoms and rhinitis following the ingestion of cyclooxygenase-1 inhibitors such as aspirin and nonselective nonsteroidal antiinflammatory drugs. Unlike allergic asthma, this disease tends to develop in adulthood, will persist into later life, and occurs in patients without an atopic history. Among patients with nasal polyposis or chronic rhinosinusitis, the prevalence is about 10 and 9%, respectively. The majority of patients report a poor quality of life, chronic nasal symptoms, and a decreased sense of smell as important factors.[81] It is now established that in these patients there is a dysregulation of proinflammatory and antiinflammatory lipid mediators: proinflammatory cysteinyl leukotrienes are markedly upregulated and the prostanoid prostaglandin E_2 is decreased.[82] Corticosteroids and leukotriene pathway modifiers are the mainstays of therapy and aspirin desensitization has been used with success in some patients.

Asthma and Chronic Obstructive Pulmonary Disease Overlap Syndrome

COPD is an inflammatory disease of the airways that is caused mostly by cigarette smoke and combustion products of biomass fuels. Many asthmatics smoke cigarettes and likely have features of both conditions. These patients are thought to experience an overlap syndrome of asthma and COPD.[83] To date, when persistent airflow obstruction is present, there is no test that definitively distinguishes asthma from COPD. As a result, there is no universally accepted definition of the asthma–COPD overlap syndrome. A simplified practical approach to this definition "quandary" has been taken by the COPDGene investigators.[84,85] The overlap syndrome is defined in patients with a diagnosis of COPD by GOLD criteria[42] and asthma defined by a subjective report of a physician diagnosis of asthma before the age of 40. This definition avoids mislabeling COPD as asthma, because COPD would not likely be seen before age 40.

Other criteria for overlap syndrome of asthma and COPD that have been used include a history or evidence of atopy (eg, hay fever), an elevated total IgE, smoking greater than 10 pack-years, a postbronchodilator FEV_1 of less than 80% predicted and an FEV_1/FVC of less than 70%, and a 15% or greater increase in FEV_1 or a 12% or greater and 200 mL or greater increase after treatment with albuterol.[86,87] When compared with patients with COPD alone,[84] the overlap patients have been described as a bit younger with less smoking intensity and with worse disease-related quality of life. They are more likely to have more severe and more frequent COPD exacerbations, and have a higher mortality.[88] Patients with overlap syndrome of asthma and COPD have been excluded from previous pharmacologic studies and further research is needed to identify the ideal therapeutic approach.

TREATMENT

The goals of successful asthma care have been established through global efforts[89] (**Box 1**). There are a number of barriers to reducing the burden of AIE, such as limited personal resources, inadequate access to medication, adverse environmental factors, significant comorbidities, and psychosocial challenges of aging. In addition, many elderly asthmatics show poor delivery technique, reducing the effectiveness of medication.[90–92] However, most patients can be treated successfully with attention to

Box 1
Goals of asthma care

1. Limit symptoms of dyspnea, wheeze, chest tightness, and cough, day and night
2. Provide normal daily activity level
3. Maintain normal or near-normal lung function
4. Reduce or eliminate asthma exacerbations; avoid emergency visits and hospitalizations
5. Minimize use of rescue medication; use lowest dose and fewest medications possible
6. Avoid side effects of medications

these cornerstones of asthma care: objective monitoring, avoidance of asthma triggers, pharmacotherapy, and patient education. These are outlined in **Table 1**.

The monitoring tools discussed are most helpful in securing a diagnosis of asthma and comparing objective measures of lung function with the patient's symptoms. Control of environmental influences is the second cornerstone of care. Both outdoor and indoor pollutants contribute to worsening asthma symptoms and new-onset asthma. Indoor pollutants include cooking and heating fuel exhaust, as well as insulating products, paints, and varnishes. The 2 main outdoor pollutants are industrial smog (sulfur dioxide particulate complex) and photochemical smog (ozone and nitrogen oxides). It is advisable to recommend that elderly asthma patients avoid, to the extent possible, exertion or exercise outside when levels of air pollution are high. Long-term passive cigarette smoke exposure has been linked to new-onset asthma in children and adults, as well as to the worsening of asthma symptoms, decreased lung function, and greater use of health services in those with preexisting asthma.[93,94]

The third cornerstone of asthma care is pharmacologic therapy.[89,95] Asthma is an episodic disease, the clinical presentation and natural history of which are highly variable from patient to patient and for any individual patient. Some patients have persistent symptoms and exacerbations from time to time. Others show long periods of remission, with sudden worsening with exposure to asthma triggers. Treatment protocols are based on this variability and use a step care pharmacologic approach based on the intensity of the asthma over time.[89,95] As symptoms and lung function worsen, step-up or add-on therapy is given. As symptoms improve, therapy can be stepped down. Several composite control measures have been developed to help the clinician assess asthma control, including the simple 5-question Asthma Control Test.[96] The long-term goal of asthma treatment is directed at reducing airway inflammation. Medications referred to as "controller therapies" are used for this purpose. Inhaled

Table 1	
Components of successful care for asthma in the elderly	
Monitoring	Use of self-assessment questionnaires, spirometry
Avoidance	Eliminate asthma "triggers," such as allergen exposure and home/workplace irritants
Treatment	Antiinflammatory therapy (inhaled corticosteroid) is the foundation of successful treatment for persistent asthma; short-acting bronchodilators for rescue therapy
Patient education	Provide the necessary tools for self-management including an action plan for exacerbation of symptoms

Table 2
Treatment choices for asthma in the elderly

Therapy	Effectiveness/Risks
SABA	Used as rescue medication for acute symptoms. May reduce need for hospitalization. Effectiveness may be reduced in elderly. Tolerated well; caution with unstable cardiovascular disease.
SAMA	Effective bronchodilator; slower onset of action and fewer cardiac effects than SABA. Symptomatic urinary outlet obstruction, and closed-angle glaucoma uncommon, but potential risks.
ICS	Cornerstone of asthma care. Can reduce hospitalizations and mortality. Underutilized in elderly. Potential risks include decreased bone mineral density, increased fracture risk, and cataracts. May not be effective with neutrophilic-driven asthma
LABA	Effective long-acting bronchodilator; not to be used alone without ICS. Questionable cardiovascular risks; usually well-tolerated.
LAMA	Shown to be effective bronchodilator as add-on therapy to ICS and ICS/LAMA in the elderly asthmatic. Especially useful in patients with ACOS. Well tolerated in elderly.
LMA	Less effective agent in the elderly than with younger asthmatics, especially when given with ICS. Safe agent, any age
Anti-IgE	Given to atopic asthmatics not responding to ICS or LABA and/or LAMA. May be effective at advanced age.
Specific immunotherapy	May be effective in selected older atopic patients; risks and benefits must be weighed carefully

Abbreviations: ACOS, overlap syndrome of asthma and chronic obstructive pulmonary disease; ICS, inhaled corticosteroid; LABA, long-acting beat agonist; LAMA, long-acting muscarinic antagonist; LMA, leukotriene modifying agents; SABA, short-acting-beta agonist; SAMA, short-acting muscarinic antagonist.

corticosteroids have become the mainstay of controller therapy for persistent asthma symptoms. Commonly used medications are reviewed in **Table 2**.

The last cornerstone of asthma management is the patient–clinician partnership. Patient education that fosters a partnership among the patient, his or her family, and those caring for the elderly patient is essential. Unfortunately it is often poorly implemented.[97] A multidimensional assessment of physical, psychological, cognitive, and social factors can impact successful treatment.[98] Self-management education provides patients with the skills necessary to control asthma and improve outcomes. The actions of the medications and potential side effects should be reviewed and the potential complications should be understood. Action plans should be written down and used as guidelines for daily care, including when to use oral corticosteroids, when to call the physician, and when to use emergency services.

SUMMARY

Asthma may occur at any age. In the elderly, it may be complicated by natural changes of the aging respiratory and immune systems. When asthma begins at a younger age, it is usually driven by atopic mechanisms and the disease may persist into old age. In some instances asthma may begin explosively at an advanced age; the pathogenesis is poorly understood. AIE is frequently associated with comorbidities of advancing age, such as heart disease, concomitant lung disease (eg, COPD), cognitive impairment, and depression. Unfortunately, geriatric-specific guidelines are not available for the diagnosis and treatment of AIE. However, using a multidimensional assessment of physical, psychological, cognitive, and social factors can impact successful treatment.

REFERENCES

1. Dodge RR, Burrows B. The prevalence and incidence of asthma and asthma-like symptoms in a general population sample. Am Rev Respir Dis 1980;122(4): 567–75.
2. Burrows B, Barbee RA, Cline MG, et al. Characteristics of asthma among elderly adults in a sample of the general population. Chest 1991;100(4):935–42.
3. Burrows B, Lebowitz MD, Barbee RA, et al. Findings before diagnoses of asthma among the elderly in a longitudinal study of a general population sample. J Allergy Clin Immunol 1991;88(6):870–7.
4. Enright PL, McClelland RL, Newman AB, et al. Underdiagnosis and undertreatment of asthma in the elderly. Cardiovascular Health Study Research Group. Chest 1999;116(3):603–13.
5. Banerjee DK, Lee GS, Malik SK, et al. Underdiagnosis of asthma in the elderly. Br J Dis Chest 1987;81(1):23–9.
6. Bauer BA, Reed CE, Yunginger JW, et al. Incidence and outcomes of asthma in the elderly. A population-based study in Rochester, Minnesota. Chest 1997; 111(2):303–10.
7. Boezen HM, Rijcken B, Schouten JP, et al. Breathlessness in elderly individuals is related to low lung function and reversibility of airway obstruction. Eur Respir J 1998;12(4):805–10.
8. Dow L, Fowler L, Phelps L, et al. Prevalence of untreated asthma in a population sample of 6000 older adults in Bristol, UK. Thorax 2001;56(6):472–6.
9. Parameswaran K, Hildreth AJ, Chadha D, et al. Asthma in the elderly: underperceived, underdiagnosed and undertreated; a community survey. Respir Med 1998;92(3):573–7.
10. Adams RJ, Wilson DH, Appleton S, et al. Underdiagnosed asthma in South Australia. Thorax 2003;58(10):846–50.
11. Braman SS, Hanania NA. Asthma in older adults. Clin Chest Med 2007;28(4): 685–702.
12. Hanania NA, King MJ, Braman SS, et al. Asthma in the elderly: current understanding and future research needs—a report of a National Institute on Aging (NIA) workshop. J Allergy Clin Immunol 2011;128(3 Suppl):S4–24.
13. Braman SS, Kaemmerlen JT, Davis SM. Asthma in the elderly. A comparison between patients with recently acquired and long-standing disease. Am Rev Respir Dis 1991;143(2):336–40.
14. Skloot GS, Busse PJ, Braman SS, et al. An official American Thoracic Society Workshop Report: evaluation and management of asthma in the elderly. Ann Am Thorac Soc 2016;13(11):2064–77.
15. Bousquet J, Khaltaev N. Global surveillance, prevention and control of chronic respiratory diseases: a comprehensive approach. Geneva (Switzerland): World Health Organization; 2007.
16. Eagan TM, Brogger JC, Eide GE, et al. The incidence of adult asthma: a review. Int J Tuberc Lung Dis 2005;9(6):603–12.
17. Moorman JE, Akinbami LJ, Bailey CM, et al. National surveillance of asthma: United States, 2001-2010. Vital Health Stat 3 2012;(35):1–58.

18. Bousquet J, Dahl R, Khaltaev N. Global alliance against chronic respiratory diseases. Eur Respir J 2007;29(2):233–9.
19. Tsai CL, Lee WY, Hanania NA, et al. Age-related differences in clinical outcomes for acute asthma in the United States, 2006-2008. J Allergy Clin Immunol 2012; 129(5):1252–8.e1.
20. Cigolle CT, Langa KM, Kabeto MU, et al. Geriatric conditions and disability: the health and retirement study. Ann Intern Med 2007;147(3):156–64.
21. Bousquet J, Jeffery PK, Busse WW, et al. Asthma. From bronchoconstriction to airways inflammation and remodeling. Am J Respir Crit Care Med 2000;161(5): 1720–45.
22. Saglani S, Lloyd CM. Novel concepts in airway inflammation and remodelling in asthma. Eur Respir J 2015;46(6):1796–804.
23. Fabbri LM, Romagnoli M, Corbetta L, et al. Differences in airway inflammation in patients with fixed airflow obstruction due to asthma or chronic obstructive pulmonary disease. Am J Respir Crit Care Med 2003;167(3):418–24.
24. Bai TR, Cooper J, Koelmeyer T, et al. The effect of age and duration of disease on airway structure in fatal asthma. Am J Respir Crit Care Med 2000;162(2 Pt 1): 663–9.
25. Gelb AF, Yamamoto A, Verbeken EK, et al. Unraveling the pathophysiology of the asthma-COPD overlap syndrome: unsuspected mild centrilobular emphysema is responsible for loss of lung elastic recoil in never smokers with asthma with persistent expiratory airflow limitation. Chest 2015;148(2):313–20.
26. Gelb AF, Licuanan J, Shinar CM, et al. Unsuspected loss of lung elastic recoil in chronic persistent asthma. Chest 2002;121(3):715–21.
27. Jedrychowski W, Krzyzanowski M, Wysocki M. Are chronic wheezing and asthma-like attacks related to FEV1 decline? The Cracow Study. Eur J Epidemiol 1988;4(3):335–42.
28. Peat JK, Woolcock AJ, Cullen K. Rate of decline of lung function in subjects with asthma. Eur J Respir Dis 1987;70(3):171–9.
29. Ulrik CS, Lange P. Decline of lung function in adults with bronchial asthma. Am J Respir Crit Care Med 1994;150(3):629–34.
30. Jedrychowski W, Maugeri U, Gomola K, et al. Effects of domestic gas cooking and passive smoking on chronic respiratory symptoms and asthma in elderly women. Int J Occup Environ Health 1995;1(1):16–20.
31. Van Schayck CP, Dompeling E, Van Herwaarden CL, et al. Interacting effects of atopy and bronchial hyperresponsiveness on the annual decline in lung function and the exacerbation rate in asthma. Am Rev Respir Dis 1991;144(6):1297–301.
32. James AL, Palmer LJ, Kicic E, et al. Decline in lung function in the Busselton Health Study: the effects of asthma and cigarette smoking. Am J Respir Crit Care Med 2005;171(2):109–14.
33. Reed CE. The natural history of asthma in adults: the problem of irreversibility. J Allergy Clin Immunol 1999;103(4):539–47.
34. King MJ, Hanania NA. Asthma in the elderly: current knowledge and future directions. Curr Opin Pulm Med 2010;16(1):55–9.
35. Leander M, Janson C, Uddenfeldt M, et al. Associations between mortality, asthma, and health-related quality of life in an elderly cohort of Swedes. J Asthma 2010;47(6):627–32.
36. National Asthma Education and Prevention Program Working Group. Consideration for diagnosing and managing asthma in the elderly. Bethesda, MD: National Institutes of Health; 1996. Publication # 96–3662. 1996.

37. Connolly MJ, Crowley JJ, Charan NB, et al. Reduced subjective awareness of bronchoconstriction provoked by methacholine in elderly asthmatic and normal subjects as measured on a simple awareness scale. Thorax 1992;47(6):410–3.
38. Enright PL, Ward BJ, Tracy RP, et al. Asthma and its association with cardiovascular disease in the elderly. The Cardiovascular Health Study Research Group. J Asthma 1996;33(1):45–53.
39. Raiha I, Impivaara O, Seppala M, et al. Determinants of symptoms suggestive of gastroesophageal reflux disease in the elderly. Scand J Gastroenterol 1993; 28(11):1011–4.
40. Raiha I, Hietanen E, Sourander L. Symptoms of gastro-oesophageal reflux disease in elderly people. Age Ageing 1991;20(5):365–70.
41. Rogers L. Role of sleep apnea and gastroesophageal reflux in severe asthma. Immunol Allergy Clin North Am 2016;36(3):461–71.
42. Rabe KF, Hurd S, Anzueto A, et al. Global strategy for the diagnosis, management, and prevention of chronic obstructive pulmonary disease: GOLD executive summary. Am J Respir Crit Care Med 2007;176(6):532–55.
43. Turkeshi E, Vaes B, Andreeva E, et al. Airflow limitation by the Global Lungs Initiative equations in a cohort of very old adults. Eur Respir J 2015;46(1):123–32.
44. Stanojevic S, Wade A, Stocks J, et al. Reference ranges for spirometry across all ages: a new approach. Am J Respir Crit Care Med 2008;177(3):253–60.
45. Hansen JE, Sun XG, Wasserman K. Spirometric criteria for airway obstruction: use percentage of FEV1/FVC ratio below the fifth percentile, not < 70%. Chest 2007;131(2):349–55.
46. Miller MR, Hankinson J, Brusasco V, et al. Standardisation of spirometry. Eur Respir J 2005;26(2):319–38.
47. Miller MR, Crapo R, Hankinson J, et al. General considerations for lung function testing. Eur Respir J 2005;26(1):153–61.
48. Pezzoli L, Giardini G, Consonni S, et al. Quality of spirometric performance in older people. Age Ageing 2003;32(1):43–6.
49. De Filippi F, Tana F, Vanzati S, et al. Study of respiratory function in the elderly with different nutritional and cognitive status and functional ability assessed by plethysmographic and spirometric parameters. Arch Gerontol Geriatr 2003; 37(1):33–43.
50. Pellegrino R, Viegi G, Brusasco V, et al. Interpretative strategies for lung function tests. Eur Respir J 2005;26(5):948–68.
51. Lehmann S, Vollset SE, Nygaard HA, et al. Factors determining performance of bronchodilator reversibility tests in middle-aged and elderly. Respir Med 2004; 98(11):1071–9.
52. Enright PL, Burchette RJ, Peters JA, et al. Peak flow lability: association with asthma and spirometry in an older cohort. Chest 1997;112(4):895–901.
53. Enright PL, McClelland RL, Buist AS, et al. Correlates of peak expiratory flow lability in elderly persons. Chest 2001;120(6):1861–8.
54. Buist AS, Vollmer WM, Wilson SR, et al. A randomized clinical trial of peak flow versus symptom monitoring in older adults with asthma. Am J Respir Crit Care Med 2006;174(10):1077–87.
55. Braman SS, Corrao WM. Bronchoprovocation testing. Clin Chest Med 1989;10(2): 165–76.
56. Connolly MJ, Kelly C, Walters EH, et al. An assessment of methacholine inhalation tests in elderly asthmatics. Age Ageing 1988;17(2):123–8.
57. Crapo RO, Casaburi R, Coates AL, et al. Guidelines for methacholine and exercise challenge testing-1999. This official statement of the American Thoracic

Society was adopted by the ATS Board of Directors, July 1999. Am J Respir Crit Care Med 2000;161(1):309–29.

58. Nyenhuis SM, Schwantes EA, Evans MD, et al. Airway neutrophil inflammatory phenotype in older subjects with asthma. J Allergy Clin Immunol 2010;125(5):1163–5.

59. Pignatti P, Ragnoli B, Radaeli A, et al. Age-related increase of airway neutrophils in older healthy nonsmoking subjects. Rejuvenation Res 2011;14(4):365–70.

60. Moore WC, Hastie AT, Li X, et al. Sputum neutrophil counts are associated with more severe asthma phenotypes using cluster analysis. J Allergy Clin Immunol 2014;133(6):1557–63.e5.

61. Mathur SK, Schwantes EA, Jarjour NN, et al. Age-related changes in eosinophil function in human subjects. Chest 2008;133(2):412–9.

62. Di Lorenzo G, Mansueto P, Ditta V, et al. Similarity and differences in elderly patients with fixed airflow obstruction by asthma and by chronic obstructive pulmonary disease. Respir Med 2008;102(2):232–8.

63. Busse PJ, Mathur SK. Age-related changes in immune function: effect on airway inflammation. J Allergy Clin Immunol 2010;126(4):690–9 [quiz: 700–1].

64. Donohue JF, Jain N. Exhaled nitric oxide to predict corticosteroid responsiveness and reduce asthma exacerbation rates. Respir Med 2013;107(7):943–52.

65. Bożek A, Filipowski M, Fischer A, et al. Characteristics of atopic bronchial asthma in seniors over 80 years of age. Biomed Res Int 2013;2013:689–782.

66. Columbo M, Wong B, Panettieri RA Jr, et al. Asthma in the elderly: the role of exhaled nitric oxide measurements. Respir Med 2013;107(5):785–7.

67. Petsky HL, Kew KM, Turner C, et al. Exhaled nitric oxide levels to guide treatment for adults with asthma. Cochrane Database Syst Rev 2016;(9):CD011440.

68. Fajt ML, Wenzel SE. Asthma phenotypes and the use of biologic medications in asthma and allergic disease: the next steps toward personalized care. J Allergy Clin Immunol 2015;135(2):299–310.

69. Baptist AP, Ross JA, Clark NM. Older adults with asthma: does age of asthma onset make a difference? J Asthma 2013;50(8):836–41.

70. Park HW, Song WJ, Kim SH, et al. Classification and implementation of asthma phenotypes in elderly patients. Ann Allergy Asthma Immunol 2015;114(1):18–22.

71. Vargas PA, Simpson PM, Gary Wheeler J, et al. Characteristics of children with asthma who are enrolled in a Head Start program. J Allergy Clin Immunol 2004;114(3):499–504.

72. Barbee RA, Lebowitz MD, Thompson HC, et al. Immediate skin-test reactivity in a general population sample. Ann Intern Med 1976;84(2):129–33.

73. Scichilone N, Callari A, Augugliaro G, et al. The impact of age on prevalence of positive skin prick tests and specific IgE tests. Respir Med 2011;105(5):651–8.

74. Wuthrich B, Schindler C, Medici TC, et al. IgE levels, atopy markers and hay fever in relation to age, sex and smoking status in a normal adult Swiss population. SAPALDIA (Swiss Study on Air Pollution and Lung Diseases in Adults) team. Int Arch Allergy Immunol 1996;111(4):396–402.

75. Rogers L, Cassino C, Berger KI, et al. Asthma in the elderly: cockroach sensitization and severity of airway obstruction in elderly nonsmokers. Chest 2002;122(5):1580–6.

76. Busse PJ, Lurslurchachai L, Sampson HA, et al. Perennial allergen-specific immunoglobulin E levels among inner-city elderly asthmatics. J Asthma 2010;47(7):781–5.

77. Litonjua AA, Sparrow D, Weiss ST, et al. Sensitization to cat allergen is associated with asthma in older men and predicts new-onset airway

hyperresponsiveness. The Normative Aging Study. Am J Respir Crit Care Med 1997;156(1):23–7.

78. Dixon AE, Holguin F, Sood A, et al. An official American Thoracic Society Workshop report: obesity and asthma. Proc Am Thorac Soc 2010;7(5):325–35.

79. Umetsu DT. Mechanisms by which obesity impacts upon asthma. Thorax 2017; 72(2):174–7.

80. Samter M, Beers RF Jr. Intolerance to aspirin. Clinical studies and consideration of its pathogenesis. Ann Intern Med 1968;68(5):975–83.

81. Ta V, White AA. Survey-defined patient experiences with aspirin-exacerbated respiratory disease. J Allergy Clin Immunol Pract 2015;3(5):711–8.

82. Steinke JW, Wilson JM. Aspirin-exacerbated respiratory disease: pathophysiological insights and clinical advances. J Asthma Allergy 2016;9:37–43.

83. Braman SS. The chronic obstructive pulmonary disease-asthma overlap syndrome. Allergy Asthma Proc 2015;36(1):11–8.

84. Hardin M, Silverman EK, Barr RG, et al. The clinical features of the overlap between COPD and asthma. Respir Res 2011;12:127.

85. Hardin M, Cho M, McDonald ML, et al. The clinical and genetic features of COPD-asthma overlap syndrome. Eur Respir J 2014;44(2):341–50.

86. Zeki AA, Schivo M, Chan A, et al. The asthma-COPD overlap syndrome: a common clinical problem in the elderly. J Allergy 2011;2011:861926.

87. Louie S, Zeki AA, Schivo M, et al. The asthma-chronic obstructive pulmonary disease overlap syndrome: pharmacotherapeutic considerations. Expert Rev Clin Pharmacol 2013;6(2):197–219.

88. Hospers JJ, Schouten JP, Weiss ST, et al. Asthma attacks with eosinophilia predict mortality from chronic obstructive pulmonary disease in a general population sample. Am J Respir Crit Care Med 1999;160(6):1869–74.

89. Reddel HK, Bateman ED, Becker A, et al. A summary of the new GINA strategy: a roadmap to asthma control. Eur Respir J 2015;46(3):622–39.

90. O'Conor R, Wolf MS, Smith SG, et al. Health literacy, cognitive function, proper use, and adherence to inhaled asthma controller medications among older adults with asthma. Chest 2015;147(5):1307–15.

91. Sofianou A, Martynenko M, Wolf MS, et al. Asthma beliefs are associated with medication adherence in older asthmatics. J Gen Intern Med 2013;28(1):67–73.

92. Bouwmeester C, Kraft J, Bungay KM. Optimizing inhaler use by pharmacist-provided education to community-dwelling elderly. Respir Med 2015;109(10):1363–8.

93. Radon K, Busching K, Heinrich J, et al. Passive smoking exposure: a risk factor for chronic bronchitis and asthma in adults? Chest 2002;122(3):1086–90.

94. Sippel JM, Pedula KL, Vollmer WM, et al. Associations of smoking with hospital-based care and quality of life in patients with obstructive airway disease. Chest 1999;115(3):691–6.

95. National Asthma Education and Prevention Program. Expert Panel Report 3 (EPR-3): guidelines for the diagnosis and management of asthma-summary report 2007. J Allergy Clin Immunol 2007;120(5 Suppl):S94–138.

96. Nathan RA, Sorkness CA, Kosinski M, et al. Development of the asthma control test: a survey for assessing asthma control. J Allergy Clin Immunol 2004; 113(1):59–65.

97. Baptist AP, Deol BB, Reddy RC, et al. Age-specific factors influencing asthma management by older adults. Qual Health Res 2010;20(1):117–24.

98. McDonald VM, Simpson JL, Higgins I, et al. Multidimensional assessment of older people with asthma and COPD: clinical management and health status. Age Ageing 2011;40(1):42–9.

Chronic Obstructive Pulmonary Disease in Elderly Patients

Felipe Cortopassi, PT, RPFT, MBA[a], Puncho Gurung, MD[b],
Victor Pinto-Plata, MD[b],*

KEYWORDS

- COPD • Elderly • Dyspnea • Aging • Pulmonary rehabilitation

KEY POINTS

- Chronic obstructive pulmonary disease (COPD) is a prevalent disease in the elderly population with a high morbidity and mortality that will continue to increase.
- COPD is underdiagnosed in the elderly population because of nonspecific symptoms and underutilization of pulmonary function testing.
- Clinical symptoms of dyspnea, cough, or sputum production should trigger a spirometry evaluation in any elderly patient.
- The goal for treating elderly patients with COPD is to prevent further lung deterioration and complications associated with the disease and to improve the patients' symptoms.
- Pulmonary rehabilitation and inhaled medications have a special role in the individualized treatment of elderly patients with COPD.

PREVALENCE, UNDERDIAGNOSES, AND ECONOMIC IMPLICATIONS

Chronic obstructive pulmonary disease (COPD) is defined as a common preventable and treatable disease characterized by persistent airflow limitation that is usually progressive and associated with an enhanced chronic inflammatory response in the airways and the lung to noxious particles or gases, with exacerbation and comorbidities contributing to the overall severity in individual patients. It is a leading cause of morbidity and mortality worldwide and results in an economic burden that is both substantial and increasing.[1]

Disclosure: V. Pinto-Plata has served as an advisory board member for Astra-Zeneca, Mylan Pharmaceutical, and GlaxoSmithKline.
[a] Pulmonary Department, Hospital Universitario Pedro Ernesto, State University of Rio de Janeiro, Avenida Vinte e oito de Setembro, 77, Segundo andar, Vila Isabel, Rio de Janeiro, Rio de Janeiro 20551-30, Brazil; [b] Pulmonary-Critical Care Medicine Division, Baystate Medical Center, 759 Chestnut Street, Springfield, MA 01199, USA
* Corresponding author.
E-mail addresses: victor.pinto-platamd@baystatehealth.org; vpinto@copdnet.org

Clin Geriatr Med 33 (2017) 539–552
http://dx.doi.org/10.1016/j.cger.2017.06.006
0749-0690/17/© 2017 Elsevier Inc. All rights reserved.

Prevalence

The prevalence of the disease in population-based studies depends on the definition of airway obstruction. Two different criteria have been used. One uses a fixed ratio (FR) of the forced expiratory volume in 1 second/forced vital capacity (FEV_1/FVC) equal to 0.7 and the other the lower limit of normal (LLN) of this ratio. **Table 1** indicates how the severity of airflow obstruction using the FEV_1 can determine the severity of the disease. The FR of 0.7 may overestimate the prevalence of obstruction. This concept is supported by the results of the National Health and Nutrition Examination Survey study, which included spirometry measurements from a representative sample of the American population between 2007 and 2010 and reported a prevalence of COPD of 10.2% using the LLN and 20.9% with the FR criteria.[2] The prevalence of the disease increases with age as shown in **Fig. 1**.[3] At 40 to 59 years of age, the prevalence was of 8.1% (LLN) and 9.2% (FR); for 60 to 79 years of age, the prevalence was 14.4% (LLN) and 22.6% (FR). It is estimated that 15 million Americans have this condition, but another 13 million are undiagnosed.[2] The disease is more prevalent in men and current or former smokers; but it differs between countries, ranging from 7.8% to 19.6% of the population[4,5] in well-conducted epidemiologic studies. The Global Burden of Disease estimated that 328 million people worldwide have COPD (168 million men and160 million women),[6] with an estimated mortality of 2.9 million annually. It was the sixth leading cause of death in 1990, fourth since 2000, and is projected to be the third by 2020.[7] It is estimated that the prevalence will continue to increase because of a persistent exposure to risk factors, including direct and secondhand exposure to cigarette smoke, biomass fuel, and occupational exposure[8] and also due to a worldwide aging of the population that is more likely to manifest the long-term effects of COPD risk factors.[9]

Underdiagnosis

Underdiagnosis has been shown to be prevalent in population and clinical studies. Talamo and colleagues[10] reported a 6.9% to 18.2% prevalence of COPD underdiagnoses in 5 Latin American countries. A worldwide study (44 sites from 27 countries) determined that the COPD prevalence ranged between 3.6% and 19.0%, and only 26% of the cases had a previous spirometry test.[11] These numbers are similar to reports of clinical studies. Damarla and colleagues[12] found that 31% of patients admitted to an acute care facility with the diagnosis of COPD had a confirmatory spirometry.

Table 1 Spirometric classification of chronic obstructive pulmonary disease severity based on postbronchodilator forced expiratory volume in 1 second	
Stage	**Spirometric Findings**
Mild	FEV_1/FVC <0.70 FEV_1 ≥80% predict
Moderate	FEV_1/FVC <0.70 50% ≤FEV_1 <80% predict
Severe	FEV_1/FVC <0.70 30% ≤FEV_1 ≤50% predict
Very severe	FEV_1/FVC <0.70 FEV_1 ≤30% predict

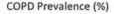

COPD Prevalence (%)

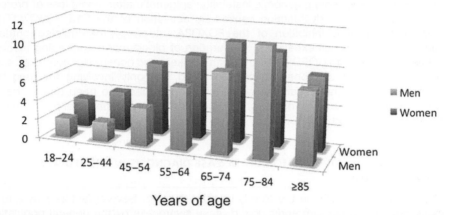

Years of age

Fig. 1. Prevalence of COPD among adults in the United States by age group and sex from 2007 to 2009.

Economic Implication

In the United States, the cost of COPD is staggering. The estimated direct cost is $29.5 billion and indirect is $20.4 billion, with one-third of the cost due to COPD exacerbations.[1] It also accounts for one-fifth of all the hospitalizations in individuals aged 75 years and older[13] and ranked second, behind ischemic heart disease, as the most frequent cause of disability-adjusted life years in the United States in 2010.[14]

LUNG PHYSIOLOGIC CHANGES IN AGING

Aging of the lung is associated with detrimental changes in ventilatory capacity, gas distribution, and gas transfer. It seems that the main factor associated with these changes is the loss of lung elastic recoil, with the concomitant increase in the mean alveolar diameter and volume and reduction in the forced expiratory flow at low lung volumes. Other contributing elements are a reduction in the power of the respiratory muscles and an increased rigidity of the chest cage. These changes are noted in the third decade of life and continue to progress throughout life.[15]

Aging and Chronic Obstructive Pulmonary Disease

Aging is defined as the progressive decline of homeostasis that occurs after the reproductive phase of life is complete leading to as increasing risk of disease or death. As described by Kirkwood,[16] aging could result from the accumulation of unrepaired cellular and molecular damage through evolved limitation in somatic maintenance and repair functions. The damage accumulates throughout life and is controlled primarily by genes. But the cellular and molecular aging is strongly influenced by chance and the failure of the organ or cell maintenance or repair that results from the integrated actions of genes, environment, and intrinsic factors. Cigarette smoke increases oxidative stress, and this causes DNA damage and accelerated aging (free radical theory of aging[17]). It is also associated with chronic inflammation that has been found in patients with COPD and also other associated comorbidities.[18] Therefore, COPD can be viewed as a disease of accelerated lung aging, with cigarette smoke or noxious environmental gases being the responsible factors that accelerate the age of the lung. Aging-related events may be worsened by several factors: telomere shortening; genomic instability; epigenetic alterations; loss of proteostasis; mitochondrial dysfunction caused by activation of the P13 K/AKT/MTOR aging pathway and inhibition of the FOXO3A/autophagy; deregulated nutrient sensing; and stem cell exhaustion.[19] Alteration of blood markers of aging mechanisms in patients with COPD compared with smokers and nonsmoker controls[20] supports the concept of global accelerated aging, not only involving the lung but probably several other organs as well. This concept has also been demonstrated with comorbidities, such as osteoporosis and early onset of stiffness of peripheral arteries in patients with COPD.[21]

CHRONIC OBSTRUCTIVE PULMONARY DISEASE DIAGNOSIS IN THE ELDERLY
Clinical Symptoms

The diagnosis of COPD in the elderly is often delayed. Several factors play a role, including nonspecific symptoms, low disease awareness by the general population and physicians, and limited use of spirometry, especially at the primary care level.[7] Most patients have an underlying history of smoking, although never smokers may constitute as many as one-fourth to one-third of COPD cases.[22] Other risk factors include a previous diagnosis of asthma, lower education level, occupational dust, chemicals fumes, biomass combustion exposure, and outdoor air pollution.

Dyspnea is a prevalent symptom in the elderly. It is frequently attributed to other comorbidities (congestive heart failure, obesity) or the natural process of aging. A common scenario is a patient who reduces physical activities because of frailty or one who limits exertion to avoid becoming dyspneic. This reduced activity results in subsequent deconditioning and a further increase in the level of breathing discomfort with activities. The evaluation of dyspnea particularly in the elderly is complex, and a careful stepwise approach is required to reach a definitive diagnosis.[23] However, it is important to quantify the amount of dyspnea; a simple and commonly used scale is the modified Medical Research Council (mMRC) scale (**Table 2**). Other COPD symptoms (cough and sputum production) are also nonspecific as they are present in asthma and lower respiratory tract infection. The lack of specific symptoms in patients with or without obvious risk factors requires a confirmatory test to make a correct diagnosis.

Table 2	
The modified Medical Research Council dyspnea scale	
Grade of Dyspnea	**Description**
0	Not troubled with breathlessness except with strenuous exercise
1	Troubled by shortness of breath when hurrying on the level or walking up a slight hill
2	Walks slower than people of the same age on the level because of breathlessness or has to stop for breath when walking at own pace on the level
3	Stops for breath after walking about 100 yd or after a few minutes on the level
4	Too breathless to leave the house or breathless when dressing or undressing

From the Global Strategy for the Diagnosis, Management and Prevention of COPD, Global Initiative for Chronic Obstructive Lung Disease (GOLD) 2017; with permission. Available from: http://goldcopd.org.

Laboratory Test

Measurement of lung function is required to confirm the diagnosis of COPD in the elderly and determine its severity. This measurement is supported by several guidelines and medical societies, including the Global Initiative for Chronic Obstructive Lung Disease (GOLD),[1] American Thoracic Society (ATS), European Respiratory Society (ERS), American College of Chest Physicians, and American College of Physicians.[24,25] The key element is the presence of a reduced ratio (FEV_1/FVC) to establish the presence of expiratory airflow limitation. The GOLD guidelines use an FR (FEV_1/FVC <0.7) to confirm the presence of airway obstruction (see **Table 1**). However, it is recognized that this ratio overdiagnoses obstruction, particularly in the elderly.[26,27] This difference is likely related to the reduction in lung elastic recoil associated with aging (see earlier section on lung physiologic changes in aging). A potential solution is to define airway obstruction as the FEV_1/FVC in the lowest 5% of the reference population (LLN) as proposed by the ATS and ERS[28] or by the LLN calculated by the lambda-mu-sigma method.[27] Recent studies have demonstrated the difference between these methods. Turkeshi and colleagues[29] studied 411 adults older than 80 years and showed that 9.2% of the patients had airway obstruction using reference values from the LLN Global Lung Initiative and 27% using the FR, without a good agreement (kappa coefficient $\leq$0.40). The airflow limitation by LLN was independently associated with mortality. However, it is unclear which one of these methods is the most appropriate, due to insufficient clinical studies comparing them, the LLN dependence on the reference equation used, and the lack of validating longitudinal studies.[1] Therefore, it seems prudent in the elderly population to use an LLN method with appropriate reference values (one that includes an elderly population) to diagnose obstructive lung disease until the GOLD committee or a respiratory society provides a definitive guideline. It is also important to remember that despite the need to confirm the diagnosis with spirometry, elderly patients with cognitive and physical impairment may not perform a valid test. Clinical judgment will dictate treatment in this particular group.

Other lung function tests include lung volumes and diffusion capacity (diffusing capacity of the lungs for carbon monoxide [DLCO]). They complement the information provided by the spirometry and are useful to explain exercise limitation related to dynamic hyperinflation and/or exercised-induced hypoxemia. The presence of hyperinflation measured by a reduced ratio of inspiratory capacity/total lung capacity (IC/TLC) is associated with survival; those patients with a reduced ratio of IC/TLC (<0.25) have a worse survival than those with a ratio more than 0.25.[30] There is evidence that bronchodilators may reduce the level of hyperinflation and improve exercise capacity.[31] The presence of a reduced diffusion capacity test should trigger an evaluation for resting and/or exercise-induced hypoxemia. It may also suggest the presence of pulmonary hypertension.

Patients with reduced DLCO or exercise-induced dyspnea should perform a 6-minute walk test (6MWT). This test is easy to obtain, with guidelines for performance and interpretation.[32] It provides additional and important information, as a shorter distance is associated with increased risk of hospitalization and mortality.[33,34] A more complete tool to identify disease severity is the composite score, BODE index[35] It combines measures of the body mass index, the level of dyspnea level, spirometry, and the walk test distance and predicts survival and health care utilization better than any of its components. **Box 1** lists several elements that also capture the severity of the disease in addition to the spirometry results. Several of them are also predictors of patient-centered outcomes.

> **Box 1**
> **Criteria to evaluate disease impact**
>
> *COPD criteria for disease impact*
> - Exacerbation per year (0–1/year and ≥2/year)
> - Exacerbation severity (outpatient treatment vs hospitalization)
> - Dyspnea scale (mMRC)
> - CAT score: less than 10 or ≥10
> - Hyperinflation (IC/TLC ≤0.25)
> - 6MWT (<350 m)
> - BODE score by quartile
>
> *Abbreviation:* CAT, COPD Assessment Test.

Radiology Evaluation

The use of chest computed tomography scan in the evaluation of elderly patients with COPD has clinical value. It is currently recommended by multiple societies as a valid lung cancer screening tool in patients aged 55 to 74 years, with 30 pack-year or greater smoking history in either a current or former smoker.[36] Several epidemiologic studies and lung cancer screening trials have shown a 2- to 4-fold increase in lung cancer risk in patients with COPD in comparison with non-COPD smokers. This risk seems to be related to the presence of emphysema, making this group of patients a particular target for effective lung cancer screening.[37] It is also used to determine an emphysema phenotype. Patients who remain symptomatic despite maximal medical therapy and have upper lobe–predominant emphysema might be candidates for surgical or nonsurgical lung volume reduction.

CHRONIC OBSTRUCTIVE PULMONARY DISEASE EXACERBATION

It is defined as a sustained worsening of the patients' condition from the normal day-to-day variation that is acute and requires change in regular medications.[38] Symptoms include increase in dyspnea or sputum volume or change in color. It is triggered by viral or bacterial infections or both but also environmental pollutants and unknown factors. Patients who require admission to the hospital usually manifest severe dyspnea, evidence of worsening hyperinflation with gas trapping and reduced expiratory flow[39,40] and show evidence of systemic inflammation[41] that correlates with the dyspnea and abnormal lung function. There is also a worsening of ventilation/perfusion mismatch resulting in need for supplemental oxyen.[42] COPD exacerbations are often recurrent[43] and have a negative impact on a patients' well-being that results in worsening of the BODE index even up to 2 years after an exacerbation.[44] Reduced survival is influenced by the number of such episodes.[45] It is, therefore, important to determine during outpatient visits the number and severity (hospitalizations) of previous exacerbations, as it will influence therapeutic interventions (medication and pulmonary rehabilitation).

MANAGEMENT AND TREATMENT OF CHRONIC OBSTRUCTIVE PULMONARY DISEASE IN ELDERLY PATIENTS

Treatment of COPD is directed toward disease prevention (smoking cessation, vaccination, and pulmonary rehabilitation), a reduction of symptoms, improvement in exercise capacity and quality of life, and decreasing the frequency and intensity of exacerbations. In patients with severe disease and/or multiple comorbidities, a discussion of goals of care and a palliative care (PC) consultation are important.

Smoking Cessation

Smoking cessation is an essential intervention because it can influence the natural history of the disease and improve survival. It is estimated that almost 1 in 5 deaths are associated with cigarette smoking, and interventions for smoking cessation are likely to reduce other comorbidities related to cigarette use. A meta-analysis that included more than 13,000 smokers with the diagnosis of COPD concluded that the use of varenicline and sublingual nicotine tablets increased the quit rate over placebo (risk ratio 2.6; confidence interval 1.29–5.24).[46] The combination of pharmacotherapy and behavioral treatment is the best effective combination to help this population to quit.

Vaccination

Influenza vaccination may reduce complications associated with lower respiratory infections and mortality. The use of influenza vaccine reduced the incidence of influenza-related acute respiratory illness (ARI) in a vaccinated group of patients with COPD irrespective of the disease severity compared with the placebo group but does not prevent other ARIs unrelated to influenza.[47] There is also evidence of a mortality reduction in patients who receive the influenza vaccine.[48] *Streptococcus pneumoniae* affects a high proportion of individual patients with COPD; vaccination is recommended, although randomized control trials have not shown a clear benefit.[49] There are 2 vaccines available: 23-valent pneumococcal polysaccharide vaccine and a newer 7-valent diphtheria-protein conjugated pneumococcal vaccine. The latter one generates a greater immunologic response in patients with COPD[50] but was not associated with a lower frequency of acute exacerbation, pneumonia, or hospitalization in a 2-year follow-up study.

Bronchodilator Therapy

The GOLD guidelines had suggested treatment of patients with COPD based on the level of disease severity (FEV_1), symptoms (dyspnea level using the mMRC scale or the COPD Assessment Test), and the number of exacerbations. The 2017 GOLD guidelines use only exacerbation history and symptom assessment to divide patients into 4 assessment categories (A–D). Treatment is afforded according to these categories.[1] However, very little advice is provided for individualized therapy according to age group. Probably, the lack of age-related suggestions is because most patients with COPD are elderly and no specific studies have been offered targeting elderly individuals.

Inhaled medications are the primary pharmacologic therapy used in patients with COPD. This therapy includes the use of short- and long-acting beta 2 adrenergic agonists (SABAs and LABAs) short- and long-acting muscarinic agents (SAMAs and LAMAs) and inhaled corticosteroids (ICSs). They are administered using different devices, including pressurized metered-dose inhalers (MDIs), dry powder inhalers (DPIs), soft mist inhalers, and nebulizers. Medication regimens can be complicated,[51] and the use of handheld inhalers (ie, pressurized MDIs and DPIs) may be particularly difficult to be used appropriately by elderly patients. Reduced IC due to hyperinflation results in a reduced peak inspiratory flow; this is problematic, as an inspiratory flow of greater than 30 L/min is considered the minimum necessary for effective medication delivery. An inspiratory flow of 60 L/min or greater is the ideal flow rate to break up the dry powder into particles less than 5 μm that enables them to reach smaller airways.[52] Physical and cognitive impairments should be considered in choice of a delivery device, as they may contribute to the difficulties some elderly patients have with handheld inhalers.[53]

Hospitalized and other institutionalized patients are more likely to receive nebulized medications. Zarowitz and O'shea[54] showed that in a study of 27,000 nursing home residents with COPD (65% aged ≥75 years), most received a nebulized SABA (49%) or SAMA (23%) in comparison with MDIs (SABA 15% or SAMA 2%). This study also reported that 42% of the participants had moderate or severe cognitive impairment and suggested that the caregivers recognized such deficits and used the nebulized medications that assured better delivery.

Many patients find spacers technically challenging and may prefer not to use them.[53] Therefore, it is very important for physicians or designated health care personnel to spend adequate time teaching and assessing how elderly patients use these devices and determine whether it would be appropriate to prescribe a nebulizer as an alternative delivery method.

The DPI with a capsule containing powder must be loaded before each inhalation. The blister packs that contain the medication capsules for DPI use may provide a challenge for elderly patients,[55] as they require 8 steps for appropriate use.[56] Fortunately, newer DPIs have the advantage of having the powder incorporated into the device, therefore, facilitating its use. Newer inhalers also include once-a-day medications, either single medications (LABA or LAMA) or combination therapy (LABA-LAMA or LABA-ICS); it is anticipated that a triple therapy will also be available. These combination therapies, more potent and once a day, are likely to facilitate therapy in the elderly and, it is hoped, improve compliance.

Once set up, nebulizers are easier for patients to use than handheld devices, as they only require normal tidal breathing for effective drug delivery.[57] The disadvantages cited in the literature for nebulizers do not relate to efficacy or drug delivery but reflect the need for daily cleaning and the longer time required for drug administration.[53]

Treatment of COPD with inhaled therapy should be customized to each older patient. The selection of inhaler device for these patients should be influenced by their cognitive, physical, and educational abilities; confirmation that they are using them correctly in follow-up visits is critical.[58]

Antibiotics and Phosphodiesterase-4 Inhibitors

There are few oral medications indicated in patients with COPD, and many patients prefer the oral route compared with inhaled medications. However, these treatments are indicated only for patients with frequent exacerbations. Roflumilast, a phosphodiesterase-4 inhibitor with weak bronchodilatory activity, has been shown to reduce the rate of moderate to severe exacerbations by 13.2% compared with placebo despite the use of an inhaled corticosteroid and long-acting β2 agonist therapy, even in combination with an LAMA.[59] Azithromycin is a macrolide antibiotic; long-term use of more than 1 year has been shown to reduce exacerbations, particularly in patients with severe COPD and previous exacerbations.[60]

Rehabilitation and Supportive Therapy in Elderly Patients with Chronic Obstructive Pulmonary Disease

The ATS and ERS[61] define pulmonary rehabilitation as a program in which patients can recondition nonpulmonary organs to improve exercise tolerance and exercise-induced dyspnea. These programs include an initial patient assessment, exercise training, education, nutritional intervention, and psychosocial support. Patients with COPD frequently obtain benefits from pulmonary rehabilitation programs (PRPs) that encourage increased exercise and maintenance of physical activity and restore independent functioning and reduce symptoms. Elderly patients with COPD may become progressively immobile and physically limited because of dyspnea and fatigue.[62] It has been shown that the presence of comorbidities does not limit the potential improvement of exercise capacity, symptoms, and quality of life in elderly individuals with COPD. Patients with COPD should be encouraged to take part in a pulmonary rehabilitation program.[61]

Usually, a standard PRP program includes aerobic exercises that involve the lower and upper extremities and enhance muscle strength and endurance.[61] There is a positive effect on overall health status and an increase in muscle strength by using a combination of endurance and resistance training.[63] A PRP is feasible and effective even when applied to elderly frail patients with COPD, as significant increases in muscle strength, gait speed, and stair climbing can be anticipated.[64] However, if elderly patients with COPD present with cognitive impairment or dementia,[65] this can significantly interfere with rehabilitation training and limit anticipated outcomes.

The benefits of pulmonary rehabilitation have been published in several randomized control trials.[66,67] Improvement has been documented in distance walked, dyspnea, exercise tolerance, and health-related quality of life. Improvement can last 12 to 18 months and can be extended if patients enroll in a maintenance pulmonary rehabilitation program.[68] Although not a traditional component of pulmonary rehabilitation, the assessment of physical balance is important. There are tools that can screen for general balance impairments and predict risk of fall.[69] Among them are the 14-item Berg Balance Scale and the Timed Up and Go assessment.[70] These tools are widely accepted and identify patients who may benefit from balance retraining and can monitor change in response to interventions.

An important goal of PRP is a global educational approach that improves patients' knowledge of their chronic condition, encourages them to recognize clinical signs and symptoms of worsening, and prompts preventive actions to avoid acute emergency care or hospitalization. It is helpful to have family members and caregivers receive education, especially when patients with very severe disease are provided with domiciliary oxygen.

Palliative Care

PC is a specialized medical approach to patients living with life-threatening conditions that promotes physical and psychosocial health and improves the quality of life of patients and their families.[71] PC is focused on 3 areas: the alleviation or control of symptoms (mainly dyspnea); timely and continuous communication of the goals of care to patients and families; and efficient psychological, social, and spiritual support. PC should be integrated into the usual care of elderly patients with severe COPD, particularly for those individuals with frequent hospital and intensive care unit admissions due to COPD exacerbations, with chronic respiratory failure or with severe comorbidities, such as congestive heart failure. The choice of patient is challenging, as prognosis is difficult to predict[72] and patients and their families are often not well-informed about COPD and have not been actively participating in the decision process. In principle, patients with GOLD stage 3 and 4[1] with frequent exacerbations, hypercarbic respiratory failure, and severe comorbidities should be considered for referral. The appropriate time for referral is variable and often challenging. Although implementation and the components of PC (multidisciplinary group) are not well defined and accepted, the goals are clear. A holistic approach by physicians, a psychologist, a respiratory therapist, and a social worker can offer comfort to patients and families alike.

SUMMARY

COPD in the elderly is a common disease, and an increase in prevalence is anticipated for the future. It is underdiagnosed, often because symptoms are not specific for this condition; there is limited use of spirometry in the primary care setting; and there is a lack of clinical suspicion. Spirometry can confirm the diagnosis. It requires the selection of adequate predictive equations to prevent overdiagnosis. An individualized approach to treatment is essential because factors such as patients' comorbidities or cognitive and physical impairment can influence the choice and delivery of inhaled medications. A holistic approach also includes nonpharmacologic interventions like smoking cessation, pulmonary rehabilitation, and lung volume reduction surgery. In advanced disease, consultation by a multidisciplinary PC service can be extremely helpful in defining goals of care and providing comfort to patients and families.

REFERENCES

1. Global Strategy for the Diagnosis, Management and Prevention of COPD, Global Initiative for Chronic Obstructive Lung Disease (GOLD) 2016. Available at: http://goldcopd.org. Accessed November 1, 2016.
2. Tilert T, Dillon C, Paulose-Ram R, et al. Estimating the U.S. prevalence of chronic obstructive pulmonary disease using pre- and post-bronchodilator spirometry: the National Health and Nutrition Examination Survey (NHANES) 2007-2010. Respir Res 2013;14:103.
3. Centers for Disease Control and Prevention NCHS, 1998-2009. Available at: http://www.cdc.gov/nchs/data/databriefs/db63_tables.pdf#2. Accessed November 18, 2016.
4. Menezes AM, Perez-Padilla R, Jardim JR, et al. Chronic obstructive pulmonary disease in five Latin American cities (the PLATINO study): a prevalence study. Lancet 2005;366(9500):1875–81.
5. Buist AS, McBurnie MA, Vollmer WM, et al. International variation in the prevalence of COPD (the BOLD Study): a population-based prevalence study. Lancet 2007;370(9589):741–50.
6. Vos T, Flaxman AD, Naghavi M, et al. Years lived with disability (YLDs) for 1160 sequelae of 289 diseases and injuries 1990-2010: a systematic analysis for the global burden of disease study 2010. Lancet 2012;380(9859):2163–96.
7. Lopez-Campos JL, Tan W, Soriano JB. Global burden of COPD. Respirology 2016;21(1):14–23.
8. Salvi SS, Barnes PJ. Chronic obstructive pulmonary disease in non-smokers. Lancet 2009;374(9691):733–43.
9. Mathers CD, Loncar D. Projections of global mortality and burden of disease from 2002 to 2030. PLoS Med 2006;3(11):e442.
10. Talamo C, de Oca MM, Halbert R, et al. Diagnostic labeling of COPD in five Latin American cities. Chest 2007;131(1):60–7.
11. Lamprecht B, Soriano JB, Studnicka M, et al. Determinants of underdiagnosis of COPD in national and international surveys. Chest 2015;148(4):971–85.
12. Damarla M, Celli BR, Mullerova HX, et al. Discrepancy in the use of confirmatory tests in patients hospitalized with the diagnosis of chronic obstructive pulmonary disease or congestive heart failure. Respir Care 2006;51(10):1120–4.
13. Mannino DM. COPD: epidemiology, prevalence, morbidity and mortality, and disease heterogeneity. Chest 2002;121(5 Suppl):121S–6S.
14. Murray CJ, Lopez AD. Measuring the global burden of disease. N Engl J Med 2013;369(5):448–57.

15. Coates J, Potal ICR, West JB, et al, editors. The lung: scientific foundations, vol. 2, 2nd edition. Philadelphia: Lippincott-Raven; 1997. p. 2193–203.

16. Kirkwood TB. Understanding the odd science of aging. Cell 2005;120(4):437–47.

17. Harman D. Free radical theory of aging: an update: increasing the functional life span. Ann N Y Acad Sci 2006;1067:10–21.

18. Divo M, Cote C, de Torres JP, et al. Comorbidities and risk of mortality in patients with chronic obstructive pulmonary disease. Am J Respir Crit Care Med 2012; 186(2):155–61.

19. Mercado N, Ito K, Barnes PJ. Accelerated ageing of the lung in COPD: new concepts. Thorax 2015;70(5):482–9.

20. Rutten EP, Gopal P, Wouters EF, et al. Various mechanistic pathways representing the aging process are altered in COPD. Chest 2016;149(1):53–61.

21. Sabit R, Bolton CE, Edwards PH, et al. Arterial stiffness and osteoporosis in chronic obstructive pulmonary disease. Am J Respir Crit Care Med 2007; 175(12):1259–65.

22. Celli BR, Halbert RJ, Nordyke RJ, et al. Airway obstruction in never smokers: results from the third national health and nutrition examination survey. Am J Med 2005;118(12):1364–72.

23. Marcus BS, McAvay G, Gill TM, et al. Respiratory symptoms, spirometric respiratory impairment, and respiratory disease in middle-aged and older persons. J Am Geriatr Soc 2015;63(2):251–7.

24. Celli BR, MacNee W, Force AET. Standards for the diagnosis and treatment of patients with COPD: a summary of the ATS/ERS position paper. Eur Respir J 2004; 23(6):932–46.

25. Qaseem A, Wilt TJ, Weinberger SE, et al. Diagnosis and management of stable chronic obstructive pulmonary disease: a clinical practice guideline update from the American College of Physicians, American College of Chest Physicians, American Thoracic Society, and European Respiratory Society. Ann Intern Med 2011;155(3):179–91.

26. Hansen JE, Sun XG, Wasserman K. Spirometric criteria for airway obstruction: use percentage of FEV1/FVC ratio below the fifth percentile, not < 70%. Chest 2007;131(2):349–55.

27. Vaz Fragoso CA, Concato J, McAvay G, et al. The ratio of FEV1 to FVC as a basis for establishing chronic obstructive pulmonary disease. Am J Respir Crit Care Med 2010;181(5):446–51.

28. Stanojevic S, Wade A, Stocks J, et al. Reference ranges for spirometry across all ages: a new approach. Am J Respir Crit Care Med 2008;177(3):253–60.

29. Turkeshi E, Vaes B, Andreeva E, et al. Airflow limitation by the global lungs initiative equations in a cohort of very old adults. Eur Respir J 2015;46(1):123–32.

30. Casanova C, Cote C, de Torres JP, et al. Inspiratory-to-total lung capacity ratio predicts mortality in patients with chronic obstructive pulmonary disease. Am J Respir Crit Care Med 2005;171(6):591–7.

31. Casaburi R, Maltais F, Porszasz J, et al. Effects of tiotropium on hyperinflation and treadmill exercise tolerance in mild to moderate chronic obstructive pulmonary disease. Ann Am Thorac Soc 2014;11(9):1351–61.

32. Holland AE, Spruit MA, Troosters T, et al. An official European Respiratory Society/American Thoracic Society technical standard: field walking tests in chronic respiratory disease. Eur Respir J 2014;44(6):1428–46.

33. Pinto-Plata VM, Cote C, Cabral H, et al. The 6-min walk distance: change over time and value as a predictor of survival in severe COPD. Eur Respir J 2004; 23(1):28–33.

34. Polkey MI, Spruit MA, Edwards LD, et al. Six-minute-walk test in chronic obstructive pulmonary disease: minimal clinically important difference for death or hospitalization. Am J Respir Crit Care Med 2013;187(4):382–6.

35. Celli BR, Cote CG, Marin JM, et al. The body-mass index, airflow obstruction, dyspnea, and exercise capacity index in chronic obstructive pulmonary disease. N Engl J Med 2004;350(10):1005–12.

36. Detterbeck FC, Mazzone PJ, Naidich DP, et al. Screening for lung cancer: diagnosis and management of lung cancer, 3rd ed: American College of Chest Physicians evidence-based clinical practice guidelines. Chest 2013;143(5 Suppl): e78S–92.

37. Gonzalez J, Marin M, Sanchez-Salcedo P, et al. Lung cancer screening in patients with chronic obstructive pulmonary disease. Ann Transl Med 2016;4(8):160.

38. Rodriguez-Roisin R. Toward a consensus definition for COPD exacerbations. Chest 2000;117(5 Suppl 2):398S–401S.

39. Stevenson NJ, Walker PP, Costello RW, et al. Lung mechanics and dyspnea during exacerbations of chronic obstructive pulmonary disease. Am J Respir Crit Care Med 2005;172(12):1510–6.

40. Parker CM, Voduc N, Aaron SD, et al. Physiological changes during symptom recovery from moderate exacerbations of COPD. Eur Respir J 2005;26(3):420–8.

41. Pinto-Plata VM, Livnat G, Girish M, et al. Systemic cytokines, clinical and physiological changes in patients hospitalized for exacerbation of COPD. Chest 2007;131(1):37–43.

42. Rodriguez-Roisin R, Drakulovic M, Rodriguez DA, et al. Ventilation-perfusion imbalance and chronic obstructive pulmonary disease staging severity. J Appl Physiol (1985) 2009;106(6):1902–8.

43. Wells JM, Washko GR, Han MK, et al. Pulmonary arterial enlargement and acute exacerbations of COPD. N Engl J Med 2012;367(10):913–21.

44. Cote CG, Dordelly LJ, Celli BR. Impact of COPD exacerbations on patient-centered outcomes. Chest 2007;131(3):696–704.

45. Soler-Cataluna JJ, Martinez-Garcia MA, Roman Sanchez P, et al. Severe acute exacerbations and mortality in patients with chronic obstructive pulmonary disease. Thorax 2005;60(11):925–31.

46. van Eerd EA, van der Meer RM, van Schayck OC, et al. Smoking cessation for people with chronic obstructive pulmonary disease. Cochrane Database Syst Rev 2016;(8):CD010744.

47. Wongsurakiat P, Maranetra KN, Wasi C, et al. Acute respiratory illness in patients with COPD and the effectiveness of influenza vaccination: a randomized controlled study. Chest 2004;125(6):2011–20.

48. Nichol KL, Margolis KL, Wuorenma J, et al. The efficacy and cost effectiveness of vaccination against influenza among elderly persons living in the community. N Engl J Med 1994;331(12):778–84.

49. Walters JA, Smith S, Poole P, et al. Injectable vaccines for preventing pneumococcal infection in patients with chronic obstructive pulmonary disease. Cochrane Database Syst Rev 2010;(11):CD001390.

50. Dransfield MT, Harnden S, Burton RL, et al. Long-term comparative immunogenicity of protein conjugate and free polysaccharide pneumococcal vaccines in chronic obstructive pulmonary disease. Clin Infect Dis 2012;55(5):e35–44.

51. Restrepo RD, Alvarez MT, Wittnebel LD, et al. Medication adherence issues in patients treated for COPD. Int J Chron Obstruct Pulmon Dis 2008;3(3):371–84.

52. Al-Showair RA, Tarsin WY, Assi KH, et al. Can all patients with COPD use the correct inhalation flow with all inhalers and does training help? Respir Med 2007; 101(11):2395–401.
53. Barrons R, Pegram A, Borries A. Inhaler device selection: special considerations in elderly patients with chronic obstructive pulmonary disease. Am J Health Syst Pharm 2011;68(13):1221–32.
54. Zarowitz BJ, O'Shea T. Chronic obstructive pulmonary disease: prevalence, characteristics, and pharmacologic treatment in nursing home residents with cognitive impairment. J Manag Care Pharm 2012;18(8):598–606.
55. Atkins PJ. Dry powder inhalers: an overview. Respir Care 2005;50(10):1304–12 [discussion: 1312].
56. Lavorini F, Magnan A, Dubus JC, et al. Effect of incorrect use of dry powder inhalers on management of patients with asthma and COPD. Respir Med 2008; 102(4):593–604.
57. Dolovich MB, Dhand R. Aerosol drug delivery: developments in device design and clinical use. Lancet 2011;377(9770):1032–45.
58. Taffet GE, Donohue JF, Altman PR. Considerations for managing chronic obstructive pulmonary disease in the elderly. Clin Interv Aging 2014;9:23–30.
59. Martinez FJ, Calverley PM, Goehring UM, et al. Effect of roflumilast on exacerbations in patients with severe chronic obstructive pulmonary disease uncontrolled by combination therapy (REACT): a multicentre randomised controlled trial. Lancet 2015;385(9971):857–66.
60. Albert RK, Connett J, Bailey WC, et al. Azithromycin for prevention of exacerbations of COPD. N Engl J Med 2011;365(8):689–98.
61. Spruit MA, Singh SJ, Garvey C, et al. An official American Thoracic Society/European Respiratory Society statement: key concepts and advances in pulmonary rehabilitation. Am J Respir Crit Care Med 2013;188(8):e13–64.
62. Yohannes AM. Pulmonary rehabilitation and outcome measures in elderly patients with chronic obstructive pulmonary disease. Gerontology 2001;47(5): 241–5.
63. Mador MJ, Bozkanat E, Aggarwal A, et al. Endurance and strength training in patients with COPD. Chest 2004;125(6):2036–45.
64. Fiatarone MA, O'Neill EF, Ryan ND, et al. Exercise training and nutritional supplementation for physical frailty in very elderly people. N Engl J Med 1994;330(25): 1769–75.
65. Chang SS, Chen S, McAvay GJ, et al. Effect of coexisting chronic obstructive pulmonary disease and cognitive impairment on health outcomes in older adults. J Am Geriatr Soc 2012;60(10):1839–46.
66. Ries AL, Kaplan RM, Myers R, et al. Maintenance after pulmonary rehabilitation in chronic lung disease: a randomized trial. Am J Respir Crit Care Med 2003;167(6): 880–8.
67. Griffiths TL, Burr ML, Campbell IA, et al. Results at 1 year of outpatient multidisciplinary pulmonary rehabilitation: a randomised controlled trial. Lancet 2000; 355(9201):362–8.
68. Guell MR, Cejudo P, Ortega F, et al. Benefits of long-term pulmonary rehabilitation maintenance program in severe COPD patients: 3 year follow-up. Am J Respir Crit Care Med 2017;195:622–9.
69. Lajoie Y, Gallagher SP. Predicting falls within the elderly community: comparison of postural sway, reaction time, the berg balance scale and the activities-specific balance confidence (ABC) scale for comparing fallers and non-fallers. Arch Gerontol Geriatr 2004;38(1):11–26.

70. Podsiadlo D, Richardson S. The timed "Up & Go": a test of basic functional mobility for frail elderly persons. J Am Geriatr Soc 1991;39(2):142–8.
71. Siouta N, van Beek K, Preston N, et al. Towards integration of palliative care in patients with chronic heart failure and chronic obstructive pulmonary disease: a systematic literature review of European guidelines and pathways. BMC Palliat Care 2016;15:18.
72. Curtis JR. Palliative and end-of-life care for patients with severe COPD. Eur Respir J 2008;32(3):796–803.

Pulmonary Vascular Diseases in the Elderly

Hooman Poor, MD

KEYWORDS

- Pulmonary vascular disease • Elderly • Pulmonary hypertension
- Pulmonary arterial hypertension

KEY POINTS

- Pulmonary hypertension is a pathologic hemodynamic condition defined by a mean pulmonary arterial pressure 25 mm Hg or greater at rest.
- Because of age-associated stiffening of the heart and the pulmonary vasculature and the higher prevalence in the elderly of comorbidities associated with its development, pulmonary hypertension is an increasingly common finding in this patient population.
- The proper characterization of patients' pulmonary hypertension is crucial to determine the optimal therapeutic strategy. Elderly patients will often have multiple reasons for the development of pulmonary hypertension.
- Treatment of pulmonary hypertension in the elderly must be done with particular care because of the presence of cardiopulmonary comorbidities in this patient population.

INTRODUCTION

Pulmonary hypertension (PH) refers to a pathologic hemodynamic disorder characterized by elevated pressure in the pulmonary vasculature. It can be a progressive, fatal disease if untreated. Because of the normal alterations in the heart and lungs that occur with aging and its association with diseases that affect older patients, PH is a common condition in the elderly. Early identification and treatment is generally suggested as advanced disease may be less responsive to therapy. Treatment of PH in the elderly must be done with close vigilance because of the presence of cardiopulmonary comorbidities and lower physiologic reserve.

NORMAL PULMONARY VASCULATURE

To understand the underlying causes of PH and its effect on the circulatory system, it is important to review the physiology of the normal pulmonary vasculature. The

Division of Pulmonary, Critical Care, and Sleep Medicine, Icahn School of Medicine at Mount Sinai, One Gustave L. Levy Place, Box 1232, New York, NY 10029, USA
E-mail address: hooman.poor@mountsinai.org

Clin Geriatr Med 33 (2017) 553–562
http://dx.doi.org/10.1016/j.cger.2017.06.007
0749-0690/17/© 2017 Elsevier Inc. All rights reserved.

geriatric.theclinics.com

pulmonary circulation can be modeled in a manner similar to an electric circuit using Ohm's law (**Fig. 1**). Ohm's law states that the voltage difference (V) across a resistor is equal to the current of electrons (I) multiplied by the resistance (R). The pressure difference between the pulmonary artery (PA) (P_{PA}) and the left atrium (P_{LA}) in the pulmonary circulation is analogous to the V in the circuit. The cardiac output (CO), which is the flow of blood through the pulmonary circulation, is analogous to the I in the circuit. The pulmonary vascular resistance (PVR) is analogous to the R in the circuit. The equation can then be rearranged to solve for P_{PA}. Composed of thin-walled and distensible vessels, the pulmonary vasculature is characterized by a low PVR under normal conditions, resulting in a low-pressure circuit.[1] A normal mean PA pressure is 14 mm Hg, and the upper limit of normal is 20 mm Hg; however, PH is defined as a mean PA pressure of 25 mm Hg or greater at rest.[2] The right ventricle (RV), a relatively weak muscle

Ohm's Law: $V = I \times R$

Physiologic Correlate for Pulmonary Circulation:

$$P_{PA} - P_{LA} = CO \times PVR \qquad P_{PA} = (CO \times PVR) + P_{LA}$$

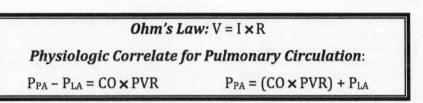

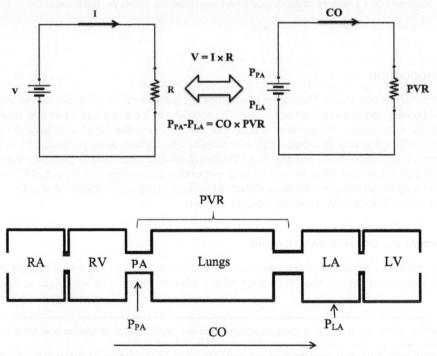

Fig. 1. Circuit diagram of the pulmonary circulation. CO, cardiac output; I, current; LA, left atrium; LV, left ventricle; PA, pulmonary artery; P_{LA}, left atrial pressure; P_{PA}, mean pulmonary artery pressure; PVR, pulmonary vascular resistance; R, resistance; RA, right atrium; RV, right ventricle; V, voltage.

compared with the left ventricle, depends on the low afterload to effectively pump blood.[3,4] Increases in RV afterload, whether it be from increased PVR or P_{LA}, decrease RV function and ultimately lead to symptoms.

CHANGES IN THE PULMONARY VASCULATURE AND HEART WITH AGING

Aging has prominent effects on the vasculature. Age-related stiffening of the systemic circulation has been well documented as contributing to isolated systemic systolic hypertension in the elderly.[5] Similar changes seem to occur in the pulmonary vasculature, leading to PA stiffening and remodeling.[1,6,7] Aging has also been associated with a decrease in the density of lung capillaries and a reduction in total capillary lung volume.[8,9] These changes in the pulmonary vasculature may lead to or accentuate elevations in PVR, resulting in PH.

Similar to the changes in the vasculature, the heart has also been shown to demonstrate stiffening with age. The resultant decrease in left ventricular compliance can ultimately lead to elevations in P_{LA} and to heart failure with preserved ejection fraction (HFpEF), (left ventricular diastolic dysfunction).[10,11] In an echocardiographic screening study, Redfield and colleagues[12] showed that one-third of the general population aged 65 to 74 years and more than half of individuals older than 75 years had evidence of subclinical mild diastolic dysfunction. This study also revealed that severe diastolic dysfunction was not an infrequent occurrence in those older than 75 years, occurring in more than 3% of that population.

CLASSIFICATION OF PULMONARY HYPERTENSION

Given that PH is defined as a mean PA pressure of 25 mm Hg or greater at rest, the equation for P_{PA} demonstrates that PH will occur if there is an elevation in CO, P_{LA}, PVR, or any combination of the 3 hemodynamic parameters. A right heart catheterization (RHC) is required to definitively diagnose PH. The pulmonary capillary wedge pressure (PCWP) is used as an estimate of the P_{LA}. Precapillary PH is defined as PH caused by an increase in PVR. Postcapillary PH is defined as PH caused by an increase in P_{LA}. The World Health Organization (WHO) classifies PH into 5 categories, group 1 to 5.[13] (**Table 1**) This classification system into 5 groups is sometimes considered to be an oversimplification of a complex syndrome. Many patients with PH may have contributions to their disease from multiple different WHO groups, a scenario commonly found in elderly patients, both as a consequence of having multiple comorbidities that cause PH and because of the age-related changes that occur in the heart and lungs.

Table 1		
World Health Organization classification of pulmonary hypertension		
WHO Group	**Cause of Pulmonary Hypertension**	**Hemodynamic Abnormality**
1	Secondary to a specific vasculopathy of the small pulmonary arteries (ie, PAH)	Elevated PVR
2	Secondary to left-sided heart failure	Elevated P_{LA}
3	Secondary to lung disease and hypoxia	Elevated PVR
4	Secondary to chronic thromboembolism	Elevated PVR
5	Secondary to miscellaneous causes	Varied

Abbreviation: PAH, pulmonary arterial hypertension.
Adapted from Simonneau G, Robbins IM, Beghetti M, et al. Updated clinical classification of pulmonary hypertension. J Am Coll Cardiol 2009;54(1 Suppl):D36; with permission.

GROUP 1: PULMONARY ARTERIAL HYPERTENSION

Pulmonary arterial hypertension (PAH) is a disease that affects the small pulmonary muscular arterioles. The pathogenesis of PAH involves an imbalance of vasoconstrictive and vasodilatory mediators, thrombosis, cell proliferation, and remodeling of the pulmonary arteries. These processes lead to the pathologic findings of medial hypertrophy, intimal proliferation and fibrosis, adventitial thickening, in situ thrombosis, and plexiform lesions, which are complex vascular lesions consisting of a focal proliferation of endothelial channels lined by myofibroblasts, smooth muscle cells, and connective tissue matrix.[14,15] Causes of PAH include idiopathic and heritable forms, drugs and toxins, connective tissues diseases, human immunodeficiency virus, portal hypertension, congenital heart disease, and schistosomiasis.[16]

The definitive diagnosis of PAH requires an RHC demonstrating precapillary PH, defined as PH (mean PA pressure ≥25 mm Hg at rest) with an elevation of PVR (>3 Woods units) and a PCWP of 15 mm Hg or less. Because WHO 3 and WHO 4 PH will have the same hemodynamic findings of precapillary PH during RHC, they must be ruled out using imaging studies and pulmonary function tests before PAH is diagnosed.

True PAH is a rare disease, with an estimated prevalence of 15 cases per million and incidence of 2.4 cases per million per year.[17] Originally called primary PH, the disease was classically described as a disease of young women, with older registries reporting that less than 10% of patients were older than 60 years.[18] Recent data from several registries have shown that the proportion of patients with PAH who are elderly is growing.[17,19–22] One recent European registry reported a median age of 71 years at diagnosis and 63% of the patients were older than 65 years.[19] The increased reported incidence and prevalence of PAH in the elderly may be caused by an aging population and growing awareness by both physicians and patients about PAH; however, it is likely that many elderly patients with PH are mischaracterized as having PAH. Because of the expected age-related changes of the pulmonary vasculature and heart along with the increased prevalence of conditions that frequently cause PH, notably left heart disease and lung disease, many elderly patients initially diagnosed with PAH may in fact have another cause of PH.

The treatment of PAH centers around the administration of pulmonary vasodilators, medications that specifically target pathways found to be abnormal in the disorder. In 1995, intravenous epoprostenol was the first pulmonary vasodilator approved for PAH.[23] Requiring a pump and central catheter for continuous infusion because of its extremely short half-life, epoprostenol is a cumbersome medication to administer. In 2001, the first oral medication for PAH, bosentan, was approved; since then, there have been more than 10 new therapies for PAH.[16] Medications for PAH include phosphodiesterase type 5 inhibitors (sildenafil, tadalafil), endothelin receptor antagonists (bosentan, ambrisentan, macitentan), soluble guanylate cyclase stimulators (riociguat), prostacyclins (epoprostenol, treprostinil, iloprost), and prostacyclin receptor agonists (selexipag). These medications have varying modes of delivery, including oral, inhaled, intravenous, and subcutaneous routes. It is important to note that with the exception of riociguat, these medications are approved by the Food and Drug Administration (FDA) for use in patients with WHO 1 PH (PAH) but not for the other forms of PH. Adverse effects of pulmonary vasodilators include hypotension, headache, diarrhea, edema, and arthralgia. These adverse effects may be potentiated by the polypharmacy often seen in elderly patients with multiple comorbidities.

GROUP 2: LEFT HEART FAILURE

Left heart failure is very common in the elderly and is the most common cause of PH.[24] The prevalence of left heart failure increases with age, one study demonstrating a prevalence of 8.4% for patients older than 75 years compared with a prevalence of 0.7% in patients aged 45 to 54 years.[12] In a study of patients older than 65 years referred for the evaluation of PH at a large pulmonary vascular disease center, PH secondary to left heart failure was the most common diagnosis.[25]

This group can be further subdivided into 3 categories: left ventricular systolic dysfunction, left ventricular diastolic dysfunction, and valvular disease.[13] In these syndromes, the abnormal function of the left side of the heart results in an elevation of P_{LA}, leading to PH. A PCWP greater than 15 mm Hg during RHC confirms the diagnosis of group 2 PH.[24]

Left ventricular systolic dysfunction, commonly associated with ischemic and dilated cardiomyopathy, and valvular diseases, specifically mitral and aortic valves, can be detected with the use of echocardiography and the diagnosis of PAH can be excluded. However, the diagnosis of HFpEF (left ventricular diastolic dysfunction) can be much more challenging, and many patients with HFpEF may be misdiagnosed as PAH.

HFpEF is a growing problem, the prevalence of HFpEF relative to systolic heart failure increasing at a rate of approximately 1% per year. Currently, approximately 50% of patients with heart failure have HFpEF, and outcomes for these patients are similar to those seen in systolic heart failure.[26] Risk factors for the development of HFpEF include older age, female sex, diabetes, obesity, obstructive sleep apnea, and hypertension.[27,28] Although a PCWP greater than 15 mm Hg with a normal ejection fraction and without significant left sided valvular disease confirms the diagnosis of HFpEF, it is important to appreciate that the PCWP is merely an estimation of P_{LA} and can frequently be inaccurate. The left ventricular end-diastolic pressure (LVEDP), a parameter that requires a left heart catheterization to measure, is a more accurate estimate of P_{LA}.[29] Performing a left heart catheterization to measure the LVEDP may be useful in cases whereby there is uncertainty as to whether the PH is precapilary or postcapillary.

Although the original pathophysiologic abnormality in patients with HFpEF-PH is an elevated P_{LA}, chronic elevations of P_{LA} increases pulmonary venous pressure, which, in some patients, leads to structural changes of the pulmonary vasculature and pulmonary arterial remodeling, resulting in an elevated PVR and precapillary PH, a hemodynamic phenotype that may mimic PAH.[30,31]

A catheterization provides hemodynamic information about one snapshot in time and may not fully reflect the patients' usual hemodynamic status. At times, patients with HFpEF-PH can have a PCWP and LVEDP of 15 mm Hg or less during the catheterization as the procedure may have been performed in the setting of a diuretic-induced reduction in blood volume. Provocative maneuvers during the catheterization, like fluid administration and exercise, may help determine whether the underlying cause of the PH is from the left side of the heart.[10,32] The presence of concentric left ventricular hypertrophy and left atrial dilation on echocardiogram can indicate that the left side of the heart has experienced increased pressures over prolonged periods of time.[33] For elderly patients who have multiple risk factors for HFpEF along with echocardiographic findings consistent with HFpEF, therapy for HFpEF-PH can often be initiated in the absence of an RHC given the high prevalence of HFpEF in the elderly.

The treatment of group 2 PH is directed at the underlying abnormality of the left side of the heart. For HFpEF-PH, treatment involves control of systemic hypertension, diuretics, salt avoidance, weight loss, pulmonary rehabilitation, and treatment of exacerbating factors like obstructive sleep apnea. In general, pulmonary vasodilators, the mainstay of treatment of group 1 PAH, are not indicated in group 2 PH and have been shown to lead to poor outcomes. These medications can increase blood flow to the left side of the heart, possibly resulting in pulmonary edema and worsening left-sided hemodynamics.[34,35] Although there may be a subgroup of patients with HFpEF-PH with significant pulmonary vascular disease that may benefit from the use of pulmonary vasodilators, future studies are needed to best identify this population.

GROUP 3: LUNG DISEASE AND HYPOXIA

Lung disease and hypoxia are relatively common causes of PH in the elderly.[25] Given its high and increasing prevalence, chronic obstructive pulmonary disease (COPD) is the most common cause of PH in group 3 PH.[36] The presence of PH in patients with COPD is associated with a worse prognosis.[37] The causes of increased PVR in patients with PH secondary to COPD are numerous and include pulmonary vascular remodeling, endothelial dysfunction, inflammation, hypoxic vasoconstriction, parenchymal and vascular destruction, and hyperinflation.[38–40] In most cases, the PH is mild, with the mean PA pressures usually between 25 and 30 mm Hg; the degree of PH is usually proportionate to the severity of the respiratory impairment.[41] A small minority of patients exhibit severe PH (mean PA pressure >35 mm Hg), which is deemed to be out of proportion to the degree of respiratory impairment.[42,43]

The initial management strategy for PH secondary to COPD, and for all group 3 PH regardless of the cause, is to optimally treat the underlying lung disease. Additionally, given the effects of hypoxic vasoconstriction with the resultant increase in PVR, supplemental oxygen should be administered to ensure an oxygen saturation of greater than 90%. In general, pulmonary vasodilators are not indicated in group 3 PH as they can worsen hypoxemia by exacerbating ventilation-perfusion mismatch.[44] In this scenario, the systemically administered pulmonary vasodilator indiscriminately vasodilates all of the pulmonary vasculature, including vessels that are perfusing poorly ventilated alveoli. Although there may be a subgroup of patients with group 3 PH who may benefit from the use of pulmonary vasodilators, future studies are needed to best identify this population.

GROUP 4: CHRONIC THROMBOEMBOLIC PULMONARY HYPERTENSION

Although the natural history for most patients with acute pulmonary embolism is for resolution of the clot, in approximately 2% to 4% of patients there is persistent obstruction of the pulmonary vasculature by residual organized thrombi, leading to increased PVR and PH, a condition known as chronic thromboembolic PH (CTEPH).[45,46] CTEPH is a relatively rare cause of PH. In most patients with CTEPH, months or even years may pass after an acute pulmonary embolism before clinically significant PH manifests, a so-called honeymoon period. The gradual progression of PH occurring in the absence of documented recurrent embolic events is thought to reflect progressive remodeling of unobstructed pulmonary vasculature because of high flow and pressure in those vessels.[47] Patients with CTEPH have a poor prognosis unless they receive treatment early.

The ventilation/perfusion (VQ) scan is the preferred method to screen for CTEPH.[48] Computed tomography pulmonary angiograms (CTPA), although able to detect obstruction in the proximal vessels, may miss obstructive lesions in the distal vessels. In one study of patients being evaluated for CTEPH, CTPA had a sensitivity of 51%, whereas the VQ scan had a sensitivity greater than 96%.[49] The gold standard for diagnosis and confirmation of CTEPH is catheter-based pulmonary angiography.[48]

The most effective treatment of CTEPH is thromboendarterectomy, a potentially curative procedure.[50,51] However, surgery is not an option for all patients as some patients are ineligible because the occlusion is in the distal vessels or because of coexisting comorbidities. Riociguat, a soluble guanylate cyclase stimulator, is an option for patients with inoperable CTEPH and is the only FDA-approved pulmonary vasodilator for CTEPH.[52] Given that elderly patients are often at higher operative risk because of comorbidities, medical management with riociguat may be beneficial in this patient population.

SUMMARY

PH in the elderly is not necessarily different than in other age groups. However, given the increased number of comorbidities in older patients and age-related changes in the pulmonary vasculature and the heart, the characterization and classification of PH in the elderly can be more complex. Treatment of PH in the elderly must be done cautiously, and future studies are needed to determine optimal management strategies for this patient population. Most patients with PH should be evaluated in a center with specific expertise in the diagnosis and management of PH.

REFERENCES

1. Reeves JT, Linehan JH, Stenmark KR. Distensibility of the normal human lung circulation during exercise. Am J Physiol Lung Cell Mol Physiol 2005;288(3): L419–25.
2. Kovacs G, Berghold A, Scheidl S, et al. Pulmonary arterial pressure during rest and exercise in healthy subjects: a systematic review. Eur Respir J 2009;34(4): 888–94.
3. Redington AN, Rigby ML, Shinebourne EA, et al. Changes in the pressure-volume relation of the right ventricle when its loading conditions are modified. Br Heart J 1990;63(1):45–9.
4. Sheehan F, Redington A. The right ventricle: anatomy, physiology and clinical imaging. Heart 2008;94(11):1510–5.
5. Redfield MM, Jacobsen SJ, Borlaug BA, et al. Age- and gender-related ventricular-vascular stiffening: a community-based study. Circulation 2005;112(15): 2254–62.
6. Hosoda Y, Kawano K, Yamasawa F, et al. Age-dependent changes of collagen and elastin content in human aorta and pulmonary artery. Angiology 1984; 35(10):615–21.
7. Mackay EH, Banks J, Sykes B, et al. Structural basis for the changing physical properties of human pulmonary vessels with age. Thorax 1978;33(3):335–44.
8. Aguilaniu B, Maitre J, Glenet S, et al. European reference equations for CO and NO lung transfer. Eur Respir J 2008;31(5):1091–7.
9. Butler C 2nd, Kleinerman J. Capillary density: alveolar diameter, a morphometric approach to ventilation and perfusion. Am Rev Respir Dis 1970;102(6):886–94.
10. Fujimoto N, Borlaug BA, Lewis GD, et al. Hemodynamic responses to rapid saline loading: the impact of age, sex, and heart failure. Circulation 2013;127(1): 55–62.

11. Chen CH, Nakayama M, Nevo E, et al. Coupled systolic-ventricular and vascular stiffening with age: implications for pressure regulation and cardiac reserve in the elderly. J Am Coll Cardiol 1998;32(5):1221–7.

12. Redfield MM, Jacobsen SJ, Burnett JC Jr, et al. Burden of systolic and diastolic ventricular dysfunction in the community: appreciating the scope of the heart failure epidemic. JAMA 2003;289(2):194–202.

13. Simonneau G, Gatzoulis MA, Adatia I, et al. Updated clinical classification of pulmonary hypertension. J Am Coll Cardiol 2013;62(25 Suppl):D34–41.

14. Humbert M, Morrell NW, Archer SL, et al. Cellular and molecular pathobiology of pulmonary arterial hypertension. J Am Coll Cardiol 2004;43(12 Suppl S): 13S–24S.

15. Pietra GG, Capron F, Stewart S, et al. Pathologic assessment of vasculopathies in pulmonary hypertension. J Am Coll Cardiol 2004;43(12 Suppl S):25S–32S.

16. McLaughlin VV, Shah SJ, Souza R, et al. Management of pulmonary arterial hypertension. J Am Coll Cardiol 2015;65(18):1976–97.

17. Humbert M, Sitbon O, Chaouat A, et al. Pulmonary arterial hypertension in France: results from a national registry. Am J Respir Crit Care Med 2006; 173(9):1023–30.

18. Rich S, Dantzker DR, Ayres SM, et al. Primary pulmonary hypertension. A national prospective study. Ann Intern Med 1987;107(2):216–23.

19. Hoeper MM, Huscher D, Ghofrani HA, et al. Elderly patients diagnosed with idiopathic pulmonary arterial hypertension: results from the COMPERA registry. Int J Cardiol 2013;168(2):871–80.

20. Ling Y, Johnson MK, Kiely DG, et al. Changing demographics, epidemiology, and survival of incident pulmonary arterial hypertension: results from the pulmonary hypertension registry of the United Kingdom and Ireland. Am J Respir Crit Care Med 2012;186(8):790–6.

21. Frost AE, Badesch DB, Barst RJ, et al. The changing picture of patients with pulmonary arterial hypertension in the United States: how REVEAL differs from historic and non-US contemporary registries. Chest 2011;139(1):128–37.

22. Badesch DB, Raskob GE, Elliott CG, et al. Pulmonary arterial hypertension: baseline characteristics from the REVEAL registry. Chest 2010;137(2):376–87.

23. Barst RJ, Rubin LJ, Long WA, et al. A comparison of continuous intravenous epoprostenol (prostacyclin) with conventional therapy for primary pulmonary hypertension. N Engl J Med 1996;334(5):296–301.

24. Galie N, Hoeper MM, Humbert M, et al. Guidelines for the diagnosis and treatment of pulmonary hypertension: the task force for the diagnosis and treatment of pulmonary hypertension of the European Society of Cardiology (ESC) and the European Respiratory Society (ERS), endorsed by the International Society of Heart and Lung Transplantation (ISHLT). Eur Heart J 2009;30(20):2493–537.

25. Pugh ME, Sivarajan L, Wang L, et al. Causes of pulmonary hypertension in the elderly. Chest 2014;146(1):159–66.

26. Owan TE, Hodge DO, Herges RM, et al. Trends in prevalence and outcome of heart failure with preserved ejection fraction. N Engl J Med 2006;355(3):251–9.

27. Klapholz M, Maurer M, Lowe AM, et al. Hospitalization for heart failure in the presence of a normal left ventricular ejection fraction: results of the New York Heart Failure Registry. J Am Coll Cardiol 2004;43(8):1432–8.

28. Fischer M, Baessler A, Hense HW, et al. Prevalence of left ventricular diastolic dysfunction in the community. Results from a Doppler echocardiographic-based survey of a population sample. Eur Heart J 2003;24(4):320–8.

29. Halpern SD, Taichman DB. Misclassification of pulmonary hypertension due to reliance on pulmonary capillary wedge pressure rather than left ventricular end-diastolic pressure. Chest 2009;136(1):37–43.
30. Thenappan T, Shah SJ, Gomberg-Maitland M, et al. Clinical characteristics of pulmonary hypertension in patients with heart failure and preserved ejection fraction. Circ Heart Fail 2011;4(3):257–65.
31. Gerges C, Gerges M, Lang MB, et al. Diastolic pulmonary vascular pressure gradient: a predictor of prognosis in "out-of-proportion" pulmonary hypertension. Chest 2013;143(3):758–66.
32. Borlaug BA, Nishimura RA, Sorajja P, et al. Exercise hemodynamics enhance diagnosis of early heart failure with preserved ejection fraction. Circ Heart Fail 2010;3(5):588–95.
33. Zile MR, Gottdiener JS, Hetzel SJ, et al. Prevalence and significance of alterations in cardiac structure and function in patients with heart failure and a preserved ejection fraction. Circulation 2011;124(23):2491–501.
34. Califf RM, Adams KF, McKenna WJ, et al. A randomized controlled trial of epoprostenol therapy for severe congestive heart failure: the Flolan International Randomized Survival Trial (FIRST). Am Heart J 1997;134(1):44–54.
35. Packer M, McMurray J, Massie BM, et al. Clinical effects of endothelin receptor antagonism with bosentan in patients with severe chronic heart failure: results of a pilot study. J Card Fail 2005;11(1):12–20.
36. Celli BR, MacNee W, Force AET. Standards for the diagnosis and treatment of patients with COPD: a summary of the ATS/ERS position paper. Eur Respir J 2004; 23(6):932 46.
37. Weitzenblum E, Hirth C, Ducolone A, et al. Prognostic value of pulmonary artery pressure in chronic obstructive pulmonary disease. Thorax 1981;36(10):752–8.
38. Santos S, Peinado VI, Ramirez J, et al. Characterization of pulmonary vascular remodelling in smokers and patients with mild COPD. Eur Respir J 2002;19(4): 632–8.
39. Fishman AP. Hypoxia on the pulmonary circulation. How and where it acts. Circ Res 1976;38(4):221–31.
40. Schrijen FV, Henriquez A, Carton D, et al. Pulmonary vascular resistance rises with lung volume on exercise in obstructed airflow disease. Clin Physiol 1989; 9(2):143–50.
41. Kessler R, Faller M, Weitzenblum E, et al. "Natural history" of pulmonary hypertension in a series of 131 patients with chronic obstructive lung disease. Am J Respir Crit Care Med 2001;164(2):219–24.
42. Chaouat A, Bugnet AS, Kadaoui N, et al. Severe pulmonary hypertension and chronic obstructive pulmonary disease. Am J Respir Crit Care Med 2005; 172(2):189–94.
43. Thabut G, Dauriat G, Stern JB, et al. Pulmonary hemodynamics in advanced COPD candidates for lung volume reduction surgery or lung transplantation. Chest 2005;127(5):1531–6.
44. Stolz D, Rasch H, Linka A, et al. A randomised, controlled trial of bosentan in severe COPD. Eur Respir J 2008;32(3):619–28.
45. Pengo V, Lensing AW, Prins MH, et al. Incidence of chronic thromboembolic pulmonary hypertension after pulmonary embolism. N Engl J Med 2004;350(22): 2257–64.
46. Becattini C, Agnelli G, Pesavento R, et al. Incidence of chronic thromboembolic pulmonary hypertension after a first episode of pulmonary embolism. Chest 2006; 130(1):172–5.

47. Moser KM, Braunwald NS. Successful surgical intervention in severe chronic thromboembolic pulmonary hypertension. Chest 1973;64(1):29–35.
48. Kim NH, Delcroix M, Jenkins DP, et al. Chronic thromboembolic pulmonary hypertension. J Am Coll Cardiol 2013;62(25 Suppl):D92–9.
49. Tunariu N, Gibbs SJ, Win Z, et al. Ventilation-perfusion scintigraphy is more sensitive than multidetector CTPA in detecting chronic thromboembolic pulmonary disease as a treatable cause of pulmonary hypertension. J Nucl Med 2007; 48(5):680–4.
50. Mayer E, Jenkins D, Lindner J, et al. Surgical management and outcome of patients with chronic thromboembolic pulmonary hypertension: results from an international prospective registry. J Thorac Cardiovasc Surg 2011;141(3):702–10.
51. Keogh AM, Mayer E, Benza RL, et al. Interventional and surgical modalities of treatment in pulmonary hypertension. J Am Coll Cardiol 2009;54(1 Suppl): S67–77.
52. Ghofrani HA, D'Armini AM, Grimminger F, et al. Riociguat for the treatment of chronic thromboembolic pulmonary hypertension. N Engl J Med 2013;369(4): 319–29.

Lung Cancer in the Older Patient

Julie A. Barta, MD[a],*, Ralph G. Zinner, MD[b], Michael Unger, MD[a]

KEYWORDS

- Lung cancer • Elderly • Lung cancer screening • Geriatric assessment
- Surgical resection • Stereotactic body radiation therapy • Targeted therapy
- Immunotherapy

KEY POINTS

- More than two-thirds of new lung cancer cases in the United States are diagnosed in patients 65 and older.
- Chronologic age or performance scores alone are not accurate predictors of patients' capacity for tolerating aggressive cancer therapies.
- Use of a comprehensive geriatric assessment to determine treatment strategy can reduce toxicities and treatment failures.
- Fit elderly patients are often able to tolerate surgical resection, radiation, and/or chemotherapy appropriate for their tumor stage, with outcomes similar to those of younger patients, albeit with higher rates of treatment-related toxicity.

INTRODUCTION

Cancers of the lung and bronchus are the leading cause of cancer deaths in both men and women in the United States and in men worldwide.[1,2] Two-thirds of new lung cancer cases are diagnosed in patients over the age of 65, and this rate is anticipated to increase over the next 2 decades.[1,3] Management of cancer in the elderly presents specific challenges, including safe acquisition of tissue for diagnosis and staging, determination of treatment strategy, and management of treatment-related toxicities in patients who have a high rate of comorbid conditions.[4] Additionally, there is a paucity of dedicated clinical trials in the elderly, leading to both undertreatment and overtreatment biases.[4] Moreover, even fit older adults experience age-related decline

Disclosure Statement: The authors have nothing to disclose.
a Division of Pulmonary and Critical Care Medicine, Sidney Kimmel Medical College of Thomas Jefferson University, 834 Walnut Street, Philadelphia, PA 19107, USA; b Department of Medical Oncology, Sidney Kimmel Medical College of Thomas Jefferson University, 925 Chestnut Street, Suite 320A, Philadelphia, PA 19107, USA
* Corresponding author. Jane and Leonard Korman Lung Center, Division of Pulmonary and Critical Care Medicine, Sidney Kimmel Medical College of Thomas Jefferson University, 834 Walnut Street, Suite 650, Philadelphia, PA 19107.
E-mail address: julie.barta@jefferson.edu

Clin Geriatr Med 33 (2017) 563–577
http://dx.doi.org/10.1016/j.cger.2017.06.008
0749-0690/17/© 2017 Elsevier Inc. All rights reserved.

in physiologic reserve and may have issues of polypharmacy, geriatric syndromes, and inadequate social support, all contributing to well-documented disparities in treatment and survival.[5] This review discusses the complex challenges facing physicians and surgeons in balancing benefits and harms in the management of lung cancer in elderly patients.

EPIDEMIOLOGY, RISK, AND AGE-RELATED DISPARITIES IN LUNG CANCER

In 2016 there were an estimated 224,390 new cases of lung cancer in the United States, with 152,220 (68%) of these occurring in patients 65 years of age and older.[1] This incidence is higher than that of the 3 other most common cancer types, with 60% of colon cancers and rectum cancers, 57% of breast cancers, and 57% of prostate cancers newly diagnosed in patients greater than or equal to 65 years old (**Fig. 1**A). Mortality in lung cancer far surpasses that of other cancers, and 72% of deaths occur in patients 65 years of age and older with lung cancer.[1] The proportion of cancer-related deaths in the elderly is highest in lung cancer compared with colon, breast, and prostate cancers (**Fig. 1**B). Globally, 60% of lung cancers are estimated to occur in patients 65 and older according to the International Agency for Research on Cancer GLOBOCAN 2012 project, with a projected increase to 68% worldwide by the year 2035 (**Fig. 2**).[2,3,6]

Lung Cancer Screening in Older Adults

Lung cancer screening remains a widely debated topic given the need to balance benefits and harms on a patient-by-patient basis while offering a screening tool that has been shown to have a population-wide mortality benefit.[7,8] Only 25% of the National Lung Screening Trial (NLST) participants were greater than or equal to 65 years old.[7] Since the publication of the NLST in 2011, which demonstrated a 20% relative reduction in lung cancer mortality by annual screening with low-dose CT over 3 years in current and recent exsmokers, subsequent analyses have shown that the highest-risk groups derive the greatest benefit from screening.[9,10] Pinsky and colleagues[11] performed a post hoc analysis of the NLST to determine whether benefit was affected by demographic factors and found no significant difference in individuals aged less than 65 years versus those aged greater than or equal to 65 years (relative risk [RR] 0.82–0.87; $P = .6$). The same group later examined additional facets of lung cancer screening in the NLST cohort by age group and found that both the absolute harms and benefits of screening were greater in the greater than or equal to 65-year-old subjects. This cohort, when compared with subjects less than 65, had higher false-positive rates with low-dose CT screening but also higher lung cancer incidence and mortality, with a higher positive predictive value of a positive screening result.[12,13] Therefore, performing lung cancer screening as part of an organized program in a setting committed to quality remains essential in the older population undergoing low-dose CT screening.

Age-related Disparities

Racial and socioeconomic disparities in lung cancer diagnosis and treatment are well described in the literature, with higher lung cancer incidence and lower survival rates among blacks and Hispanics compared with whites.[14] Similar disparities have been noted in older adults with lung cancer as well. Krok-Schoen and colleagues[15] noted on analysis of the Surveillance, Epidemiology, and End Results (SEER) database that among those aged greater than or equal to 85 years, black men had higher lung cancer incidence rates than white men and that whites had more than 3 times

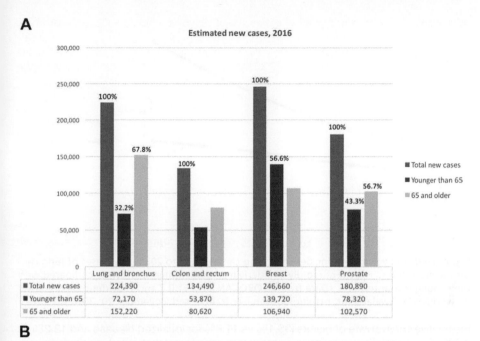

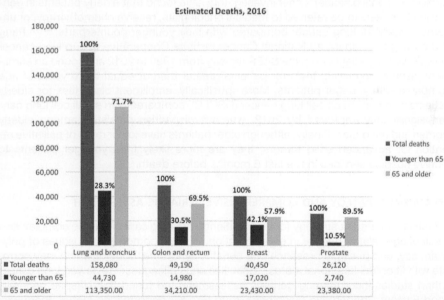

Fig. 1. Estimated (*A*) new cases of and (*B*) deaths from lung cancer in the United States in 2016. Cancers of the lung and bronchus are the most frequently diagnosed cancers among men and women age 65 and older. Lung cancer is also the most common cause of cancer deaths among all age groups. (*Data from* Siegel RL, Miller KD, Jemal A. Cancer statistics, 2016. CA Cancer J Clin 2016;66(1):7–30.)

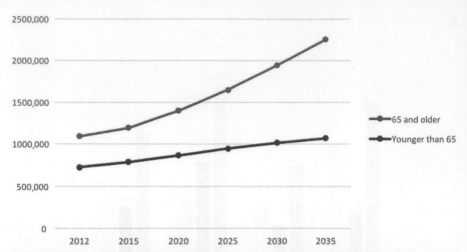

Fig. 2. Predicted worldwide incidence of lung cancer, 2012 to 2035. New cases of lung cancer are projected to rise more rapidly in elderly men and women worldwide compared with their younger counterparts. (*Data from* GLOBOCAN 2012 v1.0, Cancer incidence and mortality worldwide. Available at: http://globocan.iarc.fr. Accessed November 20, 2016.)

the relative survival rate of blacks (35.1% vs 11.6% for localized disease and 12.2% vs 3.2% for regional disease). Other investigators have found that elderly patients in general are less likely to be referred to medical oncologists, receive chemotherapy, or undergo surgery for lung cancer compared with their younger counterparts.[16–19] Pang and colleagues[20] analyzed National Cancer Institute Cooperative Group lung cancer trials as well as patients from the SEER registry from 1990 to 2012 and found an enrollment disparity in clinical trials for patients greater than or equal to 70 years of age compared with younger patients. More specifically, enrollment disparities for elderly patients with non–small cell lung cancer (NSCLC), compared with small cell lung cancer, significantly improved by 2012, whereas disparities persisted among elderly women and minorities. Finally, although older patients have lower rates of palliative radiation for advanced solid tumors, they are more likely than younger patients to receive hospice services in the last 6 months before death.[21,22]

TREATMENT STRATEGY AND COMPREHENSIVE GERIATRIC ASSESSMENT

Selecting a treatment strategy for older patients with lung cancer can be complex as a result of age-related decline in organ function, multiple comorbidities, issues of polypharmacy, and possible presence of a geriatric syndrome, none of which may correlate with fit or frail functional status.[4] Schulkes and colleagues[23] reviewed lung cancer cohort studies incorporating geriatric assessment and found that despite generally good Eastern Cooperative Oncology Group (ECOG) performance status, there was a high prevalence of cognitive impairment and inability to perform instrumental activities of daily living. Objective physical capacity and nutritional status, when additionally evaluated as part of a geriatric assessment, were significantly associated with mortality in both univariate and multivariate analyses. These results and others demonstrate that ECOG and Karnofsky Performance Scale scores when considered in isolation are insufficient for understanding fitness versus frailty in older patients with NSCLC.[24]

Comprehensive geriatric assessment (CGA) is a tool to objectively and globally evaluate domains, including functional status, comorbid medical conditions, cognitive function, psychological state, social support and socioeconomic issues, nutritional status, and medication review. CGA has been shown to predict morbidity and mortality in older patients with cancer.[4] Consensus guidelines from the National Comprehensive Cancer Network (NCCN) have recommended routine use of a CGA in patients age 65 or older with cancer.[25,26] Specific CGA tools, including the Cancer and Aging Research Group score and the Chemotherapy Risk Assessment Scale for High-Age Patients score, have been shown to predict toxicity from chemotherapy more accurately than performance status alone.[24,27]

Corre and colleagues[28] prospectively evaluated CGA-directed treatment selection among elderly patients with NSCLC in the multicenter Elderly Selection on Geriatric Index Assessment study. Elderly patients greater than or equal to 70 years old with a performance status (PS) of 0 to 2 and stage IV NSCLC were randomly assigned to chemotherapy allocation on the basis of PS and age or on the basis of CGA (when stratified between fit, vulnerable, and frail patients). Although there was no difference in the primary outcome of treatment failure-free survival, patients in the CGA arm compared with standard arm patients experienced significantly less all-grade toxicity (85.6% vs 93.4%; $P = .015$) and fewer treatment failures as a result of toxicity (4.8% vs 11.8%; $P = .007$). Patients in the CGA arm were more likely to be classified as fit (and receive a carboplatin-based doublet) or frail (and receive best supportive care), suggesting that a CGA-guided approach minimizes both undertreatment and overtreatment.[4]

LOCAL THERAPY

The current standard approach for patients with early-stage NSCLC who are surgical candidates is complete surgical resection.[29] When considering elderly patients who may be at high risk for perioperative complications, however, strategies for local therapy may include both surgical resection and definitive radiation. The decision between these modalities, and among the various substrategies within each, depends largely on both patient-related and tumor-related factors, including patient operability, tumor resectability, characteristics of the lesion(s), and patient preference.

Surgical Resection

Over the past decade, video-assisted thoracoscopic surgery (VATS) has become a standard technique for oncologic resection. Port and colleagues[30] reported that octogenarians undergoing VATS compared with thoracotomy had fewer complications, had shorter length of stay, were less likely to require admission to the intensive care unit, and required less rehabilitation after discharge. Thirty-day mortality after lobectomy for stage I NSCLC in patients over age 65 has been reported to be 4.2% in another SEER-Medicare cohort and as low as 1.19% when performed by VATS in the American College of Surgeon Surgical Quality Improvement Program database.[31,32] VATS or minimally invasive surgery has become accepted as the preferred approach to oncologic resection in appropriate candidates.

In contrast, extent of surgical resection remains a widely debated and contentious topic. The only prospective randomized controlled trial to date was published in 1995 by the Lung Cancer Study Group and reported a 3-fold increase in local recurrence and no difference in overall survival (OS) or cancer-related deaths with limited resection compared with lobectomy.[33] Although high-quality prospective data are not yet available, sublobar resection is thought to be of benefit in the presence of several prognostic factors, including anatomic segmentectomy (vs wedge resection), tumor less than 2 cm, and resection margin greater than or equal to 2 cm and for ground glass nodules.[29,34–36] Razi and colleagues[37] analyzed 1640 patients in the SEER database ages greater than or equal to 75 years with stage IA NSCLC between 1998 and 2007 and found no significant difference in risk adjusted 5-year cancer-specific survival for wedge resection, segmentectomy, or lobectomy ($P = .908$). In contrast, Shirvani and colleagues[38] examined 9093 patients age greater than or equal to 66 years with early-stage, node-negative NSCLC in the SEER-Medicare database who underwent treatment from 2003 to 2009 and found that sublobar resection was associated with worse OS (adjusted hazard ratio [AHR] 1.32; 95% CI, 1.20–1.44; $P<.001$) and lung cancer–specific survival (AHR 1.50; 95% CI, 1.19–1.75; $P<.001$) compared with lobectomy when analyzed by both proportional hazards regression and propensity score-matching analysis. Additional retrospective studies in elderly patients have shown varying results with respect to recurrence, OS, disease-free survival, and cancer-specific survival.[39–42] The ongoing CALGB 140503 trial is a prospective, randomized study of lobectomy versus sublobar resection for less than or equal to 2 cm peripheral NSCLC may provide guidance and includes adult patients of all ages.[43]

Radiation Therapy

For nonsurgical candidates with clinical stage I or II NSCLC, radiation therapy using either stereotactic body radiation therapy (SBRT) or conventional fractionation is considered definitive treatment. NCCN guidelines recommend SBRT as first-line therapy for stage I and selected node-negative stage IIA patients who are medically inoperable, decline surgical resection, or have high surgical risk.[35] Although a pooled analysis of 2 randomized trials of SBRT in operable stage I NSCLC showed similar cancer-specific outcomes and improved toxicity profile and survival for SBRT compared with surgery, these data do not yet change the standard of care for surgical candidates.[44] SBRT has also been shown to have primary tumor control rates and OS comparable to lobectomy in medically inoperable or older patients, and stereotactic ablative radiotherapy and sublobar resection achieve comparable cancer-specific survival and primary tumor control among patients of all ages.[35]

In an analysis of 3147 patients age 70 or older with early-stage NSCLC from 2003 to 2006 in the National Cancer Database, Nanda and colleagues[45] reported significantly improved OS with SBRT compared with observation alone (hazard ratio [HR] 0.64; $P<.001$). Shirvani and colleagues[38] found better OS with SBRT compared with lobectomy in the first 6 months after diagnosis (AHR 0.45; 95% CI, 0.27–0.75; $P<.001$) but worse OS thereafter (AHR 1.66; 95% CI, 0.74–1.29; $P = .94$). In an observational comparison of VATS sublobar lung resection with SBRT in patients greater than or equal to 66 years old, Paul and colleagues[46] found no difference in cancer-specific survival in tumors less than or equal to 2 cm (HR 1.32; 95% CI, 0.77–2.26; $P = .32$) and a statistically significant improvement in cancer-specific survival with thoracoscopic resection over SBRT in tumors less than or equal to 5 cm.

Radiofrequency Ablation

Radiofrequency ablation (RFA) is an ablative technique using image guidance to locally deliver frictional heating to a lung tumor and a margin of normal parenchyma.[47] Although RFA does not yet have an established role in routine management of NSCLC, it may play a role in patients who have particularly limited pulmonary function or other relative contraindications to radiation therapy. The American College of Surgeons Oncology Group conducted a recent prospective, multicenter trial in medically inoperable patients with stage IA NSCLC. In this group with a median age of 76 years, the OS rate was 86.3% at 1 year and 69.8% at 2 years with no significant change in forced expiratory volume in the first second of expiration or the diffusing capacity of lung for carbon monoxide after RFA.[47] Further research, including randomized clinical trials, is needed to clarify the role of RFA as an alternative local therapy for early-stage disease.

There are several crucial questions that remain to be answered with regard to local therapy in early-stage lung cancer. It is essential to define the roles of sublobar resection and SBRT in older adults undergoing treatment with curative intent. Moreover, additional modalities, such as RFA and microwave ablation, are the subject of ongoing investigation and offer even more options for local therapy.

SYSTEMIC THERAPY
Adjuvant Chemotherapy

Adjuvant chemotherapy is the standard of care for lung cancer with nodal involvement and for selected stage IB tumors greater than 4 cm or with other high-risk features, including poor histologic differentiation, vascular invasion, wedge resection, visceral pleural involvement, and incomplete lymph node sampling.[35] Although the Lung Adjuvant Cisplatin Evaluation pooled analysis showed a significant absolute benefit of 5.4% in 5-year survival in completely resected patients with stage I–III lung cancer, subjects over the age of 70 comprised less than 10% of the whole population.[48] No randomized clinical trials targeted to elderly patients exist in the adjuvant setting. Population database studies report similar improvement in survival with adjuvant chemotherapy in elderly cohorts.[49] Ganti and colleagues[50] analyzed 7593 patients who underwent surgical resection for stage IB to stage III NSCLC in a Veterans Health Administration cohort and compared outcomes among those aged less than 70 years and those aged greater than or equal to 70 years. The group found that adjuvant therapy, most often a carboplatin-based doublet (64.6%), led to similarly lower risk of death (HR 0.79; 95% CI, 0.72–0.86 vs HR 0.81; 95% CI, 0.71–0.92, respectively) among both younger and older patients. Cuffe and colleagues[51] examined elderly patients greater than or equal to 70 years old in the Ontario Cancer Registry and found adjuvant receipt of cisplatin by 70% with a concomitant significant increase in 4-year survival.

Locally Advanced Disease

For medically inoperable or unresectable stage IIIA or stage IIIB disease, the current standard of care is concurrent chemoradiotherapy, typically with cisplatin and etoposide at systemic doses or an alternate regimen, such as low-dose carboplatin and paclitaxel.[35] Two recent prospective randomized trials in elderly patients guide management of locally advanced disease. Atagi and colleagues,[52] in the Japan Clinical Oncology Group, randomized 200 patients greater than 70 years old with unresectable stage III NSCLC to chemoradiotherapy (60 Gy plus concurrent low-dose carboplatin) or radiotherapy alone and found significantly improved median OS with chemoradiotherapy (22.4 months; 95% CI, 16.5–33.6 vs 16.9 months; 95% CI, 13.4–20.3; HR 0.68; $P = .0179$). Patients in the chemoradiotherapy group had higher rates of grades 3 to 4 hematologic toxicity and grade 3 infection, but there was no difference between treatment arms for grades 3 to 4 pneumonitis or late lung toxicity. In an updated analysis of a phase III trial of concurrent chemoradiotherapy (cisplatin and etoposide) with or without consolidation docetaxel in unresectable stage III NSCLC, Jalal and colleagues[53] reported no improvement in survival with consolidation therapy and no difference in median survival time for older (≥70 years) versus younger patients (17.1 vs 22.8 months, respectively; $P = .15$).

Retrospective population studies using the SEER-Medicare database support these findings. Davidoff and colleagues,[54] Dawe and colleagues,[55] and other investigators[56,57] have reported that chemoradiotherapy is associated with significantly improved OS and progression-free survival (PFS) compared with radiotherapy alone and that similar OS and lung cancer–specific survival is seen with cisplatin versus carboplatin-based chemoradiotherapy in older adults.[54–57] These data suggest that fit elderly patients benefit from combined modality chemoradiotherapy but with an increased risk of toxicity.[5]

Advanced Disease

Advanced disease in fit patients has historically been treated with cytotoxic chemotherapy with a platinum-based doublet as first-line treatment.[35] For the fit elderly, 2 prospective trials support use of platinum doublets over single agents.[58,59] Quiox and colleagues,[58] in the multicenter IFCT-0501 phase III trial, showed that despite increased toxicity, carboplatin and paclitaxel doublet chemotherapy compared with vinorelbine or gemcitabine monotherapy was associated with better OS (10.3 months vs 6.2 months; HR 0.64; 95% CI, 0.52–0.78; $P<.0001$) in patients age 70 to 89 years old with locally advanced or metastatic NSCLC and World Health Organization performance status 0 to 2. There have been several studies comparing platinum doublets in chemonaive older patients with advanced NSCLC. Zhu and colleagues[60] retrospectively examined platinum doublet regimen administration in the SEER-Medicare database and found that carboplatin-paclitaxel was associated with slight but significantly better survival compared with carboplatin-gemcitabine or carboplatin-docetaxel (8 months vs 7.3 and 7.5 months, respectively). Nab-paclitaxel, a protein-bound formulation, in combination with carboplatin was well tolerated with a better response rate and OS in patients at least 70 years old, compared with carboplatin plus paclitaxel (non-protein bound) in a post-hoc analysis of patients with squamous NSCLC.[61,62] Further studies using attenuated doses of cisplatin to reduce treatment-related toxicities are in progress.[63] Bevacizumab and pemetrexed have been shown to prolong OS and PFS when added to platinum-based doublet therapy.[64] Post hoc analyses of elderly subgroups have shown mixed results for survival endpoints and often higher rates of toxicity; thus, the addition of bevacizumab to platinum doublets in older patients should be done with special care.[65,66]

Small Cell Lung Cancer

Even fewer studies exist for small cell lung cancer in elderly patients and consist mainly of retrospective subgroup analyses of larger studies.[67] The few data available show that the addition of thoracic radiotherapy to chemotherapy in elderly patients with limited-stage disease results in comparable survival rates between elderly and younger patients.[68,69] Corso and colleagues[70] recently examined patients greater than or equal to 70 years old in the National Cancer Database with limited-stage small cell lung cancer diagnosed between 2003 and 2011. They found a significant survival benefit with concurrent chemoradiotherapy over chemotherapy alone (HR 0.52; 95% CI, 0.5–0.55; $P<.0001$), with a 3-year OS of 20.6% versus 6.6% in a propensity score matching analysis.

Targeted Therapies for Actionable Mutations

There is a paucity of molecular epidemiology data in the elderly. Sacher and colleagues[71] stratified the frequency of genomic alterations by age groups among 2237 patients with NSCLC and found that EGFR and ALK mutations were significantly associated with cancer diagnosis at a younger age ($P = .02$ and $P<.001$, respectively), whereas the likelihood of harboring a KRAS mutation increased with age ($P<.001$). Awad and colleagues[72] interrogated NGS results from 6376 cancers to identify MET exon 14 mutations and found that when compared with *EGFR* and *KRAS* activating mutations, patients with *MET* exon 14 mutations were significantly older in age (median age 72.5 years vs 61 years and 65 years, respectively; *P*<.001). These mixed results were not replicated in a much larger-scale study of nationwide routine molecular profiling of 17,664 patients with advanced NSCLC by the French Cooperative Thoracic Intergroup but highlight the need for research in lung cancer genomics targeted to elderly patients.[73]

First-line treatment of advanced nonsquamous NSCLC with an activating *EGFR* mutation (most frequently exon 19 deletion or exon 21 L858R mutation), occurring in approximately 15% of lung adenocarcinomas in the United States, is an EGFR tyrosine kinase inhibitor (TKI), such as gefitinib, erlotinib, or afatinib.[35] Single-agent therapy with these TKIs has been shown to prolong PFS, objective response rate, and quality of life in comparison with chemotherapy in *EGFR*-mutated NSCLC and, in the case of afatinib, improved OS compared with chemotherapy.[74,75] Subgroup analyses of phase III trials have shown similar outcomes in elderly patients compared to the overall population.[76–79] Wheatley-Price and colleagues[76] reported no significant difference between elderly patients (≥70 years) and younger patients (<70 years) in either PFS or OS when comparing erlotinib to placebo in the National Cancer Institute of Canada Clinical Trials Group Study BR.21, although elderly patients had significantly greater rate of severe toxicity.

ALK and *ROS1* gene rearrangements are found less commonly than *EGFR* in NSCLC, with reported frequencies of 2% to 7% and 1% to 2%, respectively. Both rearrangements can be detected by fluorescence in situ hybridization and both alterations predict for clinical benefit from the TKI crizotinib, although this has not been evaluated specifically in the elderly population.[35] In a subgroup analysis, Carnidge and colleagues[80] reported an objective response rate of 60.2% in subjects aged less than 65 years and 65.0% in patients greater than or equal to 65 years old with *ALK-rearranged* NSCLC. Additional potentially actionable mutations with targeted therapies in clinical trials include *MET* amplification or exon 14 skipping mutation, *BRAF* V600E mutation, *RET* rearrangements, and *HER2* mutations.[35,74]

Immunotherapy

The most rapidly evolving aspect of lung cancer therapeutics is immunotherapy, with impressive benefits across multiple cancers, including NSCLC and small cell lung cancer. These agents mask immune checkpoint inhibitors, thereby preventing their suppression of T-cell activation, which in turn unleashes the adaptive immune response against the cancer.[35] In NSCLC, monoclonal antibodies targeting the programmed death receptor 1 (PD-1)/programmed death ligand 1 (PD-L1) checkpoint inhibitor axis are now Food and Drug Administration (FDA) approved therapy. Treatment with antibodies against PD-1, which is expressed on activated cytotoxic T cells, or PD-L1, which is expressed on tumor cells, has been shown to improve OS rates compared with single-agent docetaxel in patients who had recurrent disease after first-line platinum doublet chemotherapy, leading to FDA approvals for nivolumab and pembrolizumab (both PD-1 inhibitors) and atezolizumab (PD-L1 inhibitor) as second-line therapy in advanced NSCLC.[35,81–84] Impressively, the median duration of responses are very sustained compared with docetaxel, and these agents are associated with fewer adverse effects.[81,82]

One of these agents has recently moved to frontline therapy. In a recent randomized phase III trial, pembrolizumab, a humanized monoclonal antibody against the PD-1 receptor, was shown to improve survival in chemonaive patients. In this trial, Reck and colleagues[85] assigned 305 patients with previously untreated advanced NSCLC in patients whose tumors showed PD-L1 expression on at least 50% of their tumors cells to pembrolizumab or platinum-based doublet chemotherapy and found significantly longer PFS (10.3 vs 6 months, HR for disease progression or death 0.5 (95% CI, 0.37–0.68; P<.0001), and OS with pembrolizumab treatment. This difference was seen across all analyzed subgroups, including the 164 (54%) patients greater than or equal to 65 years old, where the HR for OS in those receiving pembrolizumab versus platinum-based chemotherapy was 0.45 (95% CI, 0.29–0.70).[85] Additionally, treatment-related adverse events of any grade were less frequent with pembrolizumab compared with platinum-based chemotherapy. This led the FDA to approve pembrolizumab for first-line therapy for patients with PD-L1 expression level greater than or equal to 50% by immunohistochemical testing and with negative or unknown test results for *EGFR* mutations, *ALK* rearrangements, and *ROS1* rearrangements.[35] The field of immune checkpoint inhibition is rapidly evolving, and current clinical trials are evaluating efficacy of combination therapy and use in earlier disease. Immune checkpoint inhibitors are being explored in small cell lung cancer with the NCCN, including either nivolumab or nivolumab plus ipilimumab as an option in recurrent resistant advanced small cell lung cancer based on phase II data showing promising efficacy.[86]

SUMMARY

Elderly patients make up more than two-thirds of new cases of NSCLC each year. This cohort is at particularly high risk for both undertreatment and overtreatment. Chronologic age and performance scores alone are limited in their capacity to predict older patients' ability to tolerate standard of care cancer therapies, and CGA is an essential part of choosing an appropriate therapeutic strategy to optimize the balance of treatment harms and benefits. With care and appropriate patient selection, however, standard or modified anticancer interventions can offer both improved survival and well-being compared with supportive care alone in all stages of disease, with data especially robust in NSCLC. This article reviews data supporting the utilization of surgical resection for early-stage disease, adjuvant chemotherapy, and, in locally advanced NSCLC, combined modality treatment in fit older patients. In addition, data support a role for standard of care treatment of first-line and second-line systemic therapies in fit elderly patients with advanced NSCLC. For frail elderly patients, lower-risk modalities can be considered, such as SBRT in local disease NSCLC, modified radiation with or without concurrent chemotherapy in regional NSCLC, and modified dosing and careful tailoring of systemic therapy for advanced disease. Ongoing research in immunotherapy also provides an environment ripe for advances highly relevant to the elderly population, given promising efficacy and tolerability.

REFERENCES

1. Siegel RL, Miller KD, Jemal A. Cancer statistics, 2016. CA Cancer J Clin 2016; 66(1):7–30.
2. Torre LA, Bray F, Siegel RL, et al. Global cancer statistics, 2012. CA Cancer J Clin 2015;65(2):87–108.
3. Torre LA, Siegel RL, Ward EM, et al. Global cancer incidence and mortality rates and trends—an update. Cancer Epidemiol Biomarkers Prev 2016;25(1):16–27.
4. Presley CJ, Gross CP, Lilenbaum RC. Optimizing treatment risk and benefit for elderly patients with advanced non-small-cell lung cancer: the right treatment for the right patient. J Clin Oncol 2016;34(13):1438–42.
5. Gridelli C, Balducci L, Ciardiello F, et al. Treatment of elderly patients with non-small-cell lung cancer: results of an International expert panel meeting of the Italian Association of Thoracic Oncology. Clin Lung Cancer 2015;16(5):325–33.

6. Ferlay J, Soerjomataram I, Ervik M, et al. GLOBOCAN 2012 v1.0, Cancer incidence and mortality worldwide: IARC CancerBase No. 11(Internet) 2013. 2014. Available at: http://globocan.iarc.fr/. Accessed November 20, 2016.

7. Aberle DR, Adams AM, Berg CD, et al. Reduced lung-cancer mortality with low-dose computed tomographic screening. N Engl J Med 2011;365(5):395–409.

8. Mazzone P, Powell CA, Arenberg D, et al. Components necessary for high-quality lung cancer screening: American College of chest physicians and American thoracic society policy statement. Chest 2015;147(2):295–303.

9. Kovalchik SA, Tammemagi M, Berg CD, et al. Targeting of low-dose CT screening according to the risk of lung-cancer death. N Engl J Med 2013;369(3):245–54.

10. Katki HA, Kovalchik SA, Berg CD, et al. Development and validation of risk models to select ever-smokers for CT lung cancer screening. JAMA 2016; 315(21):2300–11.

11. Pinsky PF, Church TR, Izmirlian G, et al. The national lung screening trial: results stratified by demographics, smoking history, and lung cancer histology. Cancer 2013;119(22):3976–83.

12. Pinsky PF, Gierada DS, Hocking W, et al. National lung screening trial findings by age: Medicare-eligible versus under-65 population. Ann Intern Med 2014;161(9): 627–33.

13. Gould MK. Lung cancer screening and elderly adults: do we have sufficient evidence? Ann Intern Med 2014;161(9):672–3.

14. Jonnalagadda S, Lin JJ, Nelson JE, et al. Racial and ethnic differences in beliefs about lung cancer care. Chest 2012;142(5):1251–8.

15. Krok-Schoen JL, Fisher JL, Baltic RD, et al. White-black differences in cancer incidence, stage at diagnosis, and survival among adults aged 85 years and older in the United States. Cancer Epidemiol Biomarkers Prev 2016,25(11): 1517–23.

16. Revels SL, Banerjee M, Yin H, et al. Racial disparities in surgical resection and survival among elderly patients with poor prognosis cancer. J Am Coll Surg 2013;216(2):312–9.

17. Dawe DE, Pond GR, Ellis PM. Assessment of referral and chemotherapy treatment patterns for elderly patients with non-small-cell lung cancer. Clin Lung Cancer 2016;17(6):563–72.e562.

18. Groth SS, Al-Refaie WB, Zhong W, et al. Effect of insurance status on the surgical treatment of early-stage non-small cell lung cancer. Ann Thorac Surg 2013;95(4): 1221–6.

19. Sineshaw HM, Wu XC, Flanders WD, et al. Variations in receipt of curative-intent surgery for early-stage non-small cell lung cancer (NSCLC) by state. J Thorac Oncol 2016;11(6):880–9.

20. Pang HH, Wang X, Stinchcombe TE, et al. Enrollment trends and disparity among patients with lung cancer in National clinical trials, 1990 to 2012. J Clin Oncol 2016;34(33):3992–9.

21. Wong J, Xu B, Yeung HN, et al. Age disparity in palliative radiation therapy among patients with advanced cancer. Int J Radiat Oncol Biol Phys 2014;90(1):224–30.

22. Hardy D, Chan W, Liu CC, et al. Racial disparities in the use of hospice services according to geographic residence and socioeconomic status in an elderly cohort with nonsmall cell lung cancer. Cancer 2011;117(7):1506–15.

23. Schulkes KJ, Hamaker ME, van den Bos F, et al. Relevance of a geriatric assessment for elderly patients with lung cancer-a systematic review. Clin Lung Cancer 2016;17(5):341–9.e343.

24. Extermann M, Boler I, Reich RR, et al. Predicting the risk of chemotherapy toxicity in older patients: the chemotherapy risk assessment scale for high-age patients (CRASH) score. Cancer 2012;118(13):3377–86.

25. NCCN Guidelines: Older Adult Oncology. NCCN clinical practice guidelines in oncology 2016, 2.2016. Available at: https://www.nccn.org/professionals/physician_gls/f_guidelines.asp. Accessed November 20, 2016.

26. Wildiers H, Heeren P, Puts M, et al. International society of geriatric oncology consensus on geriatric assessment in older patients with cancer. J Clin Oncol 2014;32(24):2595–603.

27. Hurria A, Togawa K, Mohile SG, et al. Predicting chemotherapy toxicity in older adults with cancer: a prospective multicenter study. J Clin Oncol 2011;29(25): 3457–65.

28. Corre R, Greillier L, Le Caer H, et al. Use of a comprehensive geriatric assessment for the management of elderly patients with advanced non-small-cell lung cancer: the phase III randomized ESOGIA-GFPC-GECP 08-02 study. J Clin Oncol 2016;34(13):1476–83.

29. Sun HH, Sesti J, Donington JS. Surgical treatment of early I stage lung cancer: what has changed and what will change in the future. Semin Respir Crit Care Med 2016;37(5):708–15.

30. Port JL, Mirza FM, Lee PC, et al. Lobectomy in octogenarians with non-small cell lung cancer: ramifications of increasing life expectancy and the benefits of minimally invasive surgery. Ann Thorac Surg 2011;92(6):1951–7.

31. Rueth NM, Parsons HM, Habermann EB, et al. Surgical treatment of lung cancer: predicting postoperative morbidity in the elderly population. J Thorac Cardiovasc Surg 2012;143(6):1314–23.

32. Bravo Iniguez CE, Armstrong KW, Cooper Z, et al. Thirty-day mortality after lobectomy in elderly patients eligible for lung cancer screening. Ann Thorac Surg 2016; 101(2):541–6.

33. Ginsberg RJ, Rubinstein LV. Randomized trial of lobectomy versus limited resection for T1 N0 non-small cell lung cancer. Lung Cancer Study Group. Ann Thorac Surg 1995;60(3):615–22 [discussion: 622–3].

34. Smith CB, Kale M, Mhango G, et al. Comparative outcomes of elderly stage I lung cancer patients treated with segmentectomy via video-assisted thoracoscopic surgery versus open resection. J Thorac Oncol 2014;9(3):383–9.

35. NCCN Guidelines: Non-Small Cell Lung Cancer. NCCN clinical practice guidelines in oncology 2016, Version 3.2017. Available at: https://www.nccn.org/professionals/physician_gls/f_guidelines.asp. Accessed November 20, 2016.

36. Travis WD, Brambilla E, Noguchi M, et al. International Association for the study of lung cancer/American Thoracic Society/European Respiratory Society: International multidisciplinary classification of lung adenocarcinoma: executive summary. Proc Am Thorac Soc 2011;8(5):381–5.

37. Razi SS, John MM, Sainathan S, et al. Sublobar resection is equivalent to lobectomy for T1a non-small cell lung cancer in the elderly: a surveillance, epidemiology, and end results database analysis. J Surg Res 2016;200(2):683–9.

38. Shirvani SM, Jiang J, Chang JY, et al. Lobectomy, sublobar resection, and stereotactic ablative radiotherapy for early-stage non-small cell lung cancers in the elderly. JAMA Surg 2014;149(12):1244–53.

39. Okamoto J, Kubokura H, Usuda J. Factors determining the choice of surgical procedure in elderly patients with non-small cell lung cancer. Ann Thorac Cardiovasc Surg 2016;22(3):131–8.

40. Zhang Y, Yuan C, Zhang Y, et al. Survival following segmentectomy or lobectomy in elderly patients with early-stage lung cancer. Oncotarget 2016;7(14):19081-6.

41. Fiorelli A, Caronia FP, Daddi N, et al. Sublobar resection versus lobectomy for stage I non-small cell lung cancer: an appropriate choice in elderly patients? Surg Today 2016;46(12):1370-82.

42. Shirvani SM, Jiang J, Chang JY, et al. Comparative effectiveness of 5 treatment strategies for early-stage non-small cell lung cancer in the elderly. Int J Radiat Oncol Biol Phys 2012;84(5):1060-70.

43. Comparison of different types of surgery in treating patients with stage IA non-small cell lung cancer. 2016. Available at: https://clinicaltrials.gov/ct2/show/NCT00499330. Accessed November 20, 2016.

44. Chang JY, Senan S, Paul MA, et al. Stereotactic ablative radiotherapy versus lobectomy for operable stage I non-small-cell lung cancer: a pooled analysis of two randomised trials. Lancet Oncol 2015;16(6):630-7.

45. Nanda RH, Liu Y, Gillespie TW, et al. Stereotactic body radiation therapy versus no treatment for early stage non-small cell lung cancer in medically inoperable elderly patients: a National cancer data base analysis. Cancer 2015;121(23):4222-30.

46. Paul S, Lee PC, Mao J, et al. Long term survival with stereotactic ablative radiotherapy (SABR) versus thoracoscopic sublobar lung resection in elderly people: national population based study with propensity matched comparative analysis. BMJ 2016;354:i3570.

47. Dupuy DE, Fernando HC, Hillman S, et al. Radiofrequency ablation of stage IA non-small cell lung cancer in medically inoperable patients: results from the American College of Surgeons Oncology Group Z4033 (Alliance) trial. Cancer 2015;121(19):3491-8.

48. Pignon J-P, Tribodet H, Scagliotti GV, et al. Lung adjuvant cisplatin evaluation: a pooled analysis by the LACE collaborative group. J Clin Oncol 2008;26(21):3552-9.

49. Wisnivesky JP, Smith CB, Packer S, et al. Survival and risk of adverse events in older patients receiving postoperative adjuvant chemotherapy for resected stages II-IIIA lung cancer: observational cohort study. BMJ 2011;343:d4013.

50. Ganti AK, Williams CD, Gajra A, et al. Effect of age on the efficacy of adjuvant chemotherapy for resected non-small cell lung cancer. Cancer 2015;121(15):2578-85.

51. Cuffe S, Booth CM, Peng Y, et al. Adjuvant chemotherapy for non-small-cell lung cancer in the elderly: a population-based study in Ontario, Canada. J Clin Oncol 2012;30(15):1813-21.

52. Atagi S, Kawahara M, Yokoyama A, et al. Thoracic radiotherapy with or without daily low-dose carboplatin in elderly patients with non-small-cell lung cancer: a randomised, controlled, phase 3 trial by the Japan Clinical Oncology Group (JCOG0301). Lancet Oncol 2012;13(7):671-8.

53. Jalal SI, Riggs HD, Melnyk A, et al. Updated survival and outcomes for older adults with inoperable stage III non-small-cell lung cancer treated with cisplatin, etoposide, and concurrent chest radiation with or without consolidation docetaxel: analysis of a phase III trial from the Hoosier Oncology Group (HOG) and US Oncology. Ann Oncol 2011;23(7):1730-8.

54. Davidoff AJ, Gardner JF, Seal B, et al. Population-based estimates of survival benefit associated with combined modality therapy in elderly patients with locally advanced non-small cell lung cancer. J Thorac Oncol 2011;6(5):934-41.

55. Dawe DE, Christiansen D, Swaminath A, et al. Chemoradiotherapy versus radiotherapy alone in elderly patients with stage III non-small cell lung cancer: a systematic review and meta-analysis. Lung Cancer 2016;99:180–5.

56. Ezer N, Smith CB, Galsky MD, et al. Cisplatin vs. carboplatin-based chemoradiotherapy in patients >65 years of age with stage III non-small cell lung cancer. Radiother Oncol 2014;112(2):272–8.

57. Sigel K, Lurslurchachai L, Bonomi M, et al. Effectiveness of radiation therapy alone for elderly patients with unresected stage III non-small cell lung cancer. Lung Cancer 2013;82(2):266–70.

58. Quoix E, Zalcman G, Oster JP, et al. Carboplatin and weekly paclitaxel doublet chemotherapy compared with monotherapy in elderly patients with advanced non-small-cell lung cancer: IFCT-0501 randomised, phase 3 trial. Lancet 2011; 378(9796):1079–88.

59. Abe T, Takeda K, Ohe Y, et al. Randomized phase III trial comparing weekly docetaxel plus cisplatin versus docetaxel monotherapy every 3 weeks in elderly patients with advanced non-small-cell lung cancer: the intergroup trial JCOG0803/WJOG4307L. J Clin Oncol 2015;33(6):575–81.

60. Zhu J, Sharma DB, Chen AB, et al. Comparative effectiveness of three platinum-doublet chemotherapy regimens in elderly patients with advanced non-small cell lung cancer. Cancer 2013;119(11):2048–60.

61. Socinski MA, Langer CJ, Okamoto I, et al. Safety and efficacy of weekly nab(R)-paclitaxel in combination with carboplatin as first-line therapy in elderly patients with advanced non-small-cell lung cancer. Ann Oncol 2013;24(2):314–21.

62. Gridelli C, Chen T, Ko A, et al. P1.48: nab-Paclitaxel + Carboplatin in advanced non-small cell lung cancer: outcomes in elderly patients with squamous histology: track: advanced NSCLC. J Thorac Oncol 2016;11(10S):S213.

63. Gridelli C, Rossi A, Di Maio M, et al. Rationale and design of MILES-3 and MILES-4 studies: two randomized phase 3 trials comparing single-agent chemotherapy versus cisplatin-based doublets in elderly patients with advanced non-small-cell lung cancer. Clin Lung Cancer 2014;15(2):166–70.

64. Gridelli C, de Marinis F, Thomas M, et al. Final efficacy and safety results of pemetrexed continuation maintenance therapy in the elderly from the PARAMOUNT phase III study. J Thorac Oncol 2014;9(7):991–7.

65. Zhu J, Sharma DB, Gray SW, et al. Carboplatin and paclitaxel with vs without bevacizumab in older patients with advanced non-small cell lung cancer. JAMA 2012;307(15):1593–601.

66. Langer CJ, Socinski MA, Patel JD, et al. Isolating the role of Bevacizumab in elderly patients with previously untreated nonsquamous non-small cell lung cancer: secondary analyses of the ECOG 4599 and pointbreak trials. Am J Clin Oncol 2016;39(5):441–7.

67. Gridelli C, Casaluce F, Sgambato A, et al. Treatment of limited-stage small cell lung cancer in the elderly, chemotherapy vs. sequential chemoradiotherapy vs. concurrent chemoradiotherapy: that's the question. Transl Lung Cancer Res 2016;5(2):150–4.

68. Schild SE, Stella PJ, Brooks BJ, et al. Results of combined-modality therapy for limited-stage small cell lung carcinoma in the elderly. Cancer 2005;103(11): 2349–54.

69. Yuen AR, Zou G, Turrisi AT, et al. Similar outcome of elderly patients in intergroup trial 0096: cisplatin, etoposide, and thoracic radiotherapy administered once or twice daily in limited stage small cell lung carcinoma. Cancer 2000;89(9): 1953–60.

70. Corso CD, Rutter CE, Park HS, et al. Role of chemoradiotherapy in elderly patients with limited-stage small-cell lung cancer. J Clin Oncol 2015;33(36):4240–6.

71. Sacher AG, Dahlberg SE, Heng J, et al. Association between younger age and targetable genomic alterations and prognosis in non–small-cell lung cancer. JAMA Oncol 2016;2(3):313–20.

72. Awad MM, Oxnard GR, Jackman DM, et al. MET Exon 14 mutations in non–small-cell lung cancer are associated with advanced age and stage-dependent MET genomic amplification and c-Met overexpression. J Clin Oncol 2016;34(7): 721–30.

73. Barlesi F, Mazieres J, Merlio JP, et al. Routine molecular profiling of patients with advanced non-small-cell lung cancer: results of a 1-year nationwide programme of the French Cooperative Thoracic Intergroup (IFCT). Lancet 2016;387(10026): 1415–26.

74. Hirsch FR, Scagliotti GV, Mulshine JL, et al. Lung cancer: current therapies and new targeted treatments. Lancet 2017;389(10066):299–311.

75. Yang JC, Wu YL, Schuler M, et al. Afatinib versus cisplatin-based chemotherapy for EGFR mutation-positive lung adenocarcinoma (LUX-Lung 3 and LUX-Lung 6): analysis of overall survival data from two randomised, phase 3 trials. Lancet Oncol 2015;16(2):141–51.

76. Wheatley-Price P, Ding K, Seymour L, et al. Erlotinib for advanced non–small-cell lung cancer in the elderly: an analysis of the National Cancer Institute of Canada clinical trials group study BR.21. J Clin Oncol 2008;26(14):2350–7.

77. Fein L, Wu Y-L, Sequist LV, et al. P1.33: afatinib versus chemotherapy for EGFR mutation-positive NSCLC patients aged ≥ 65 years: subgroup analysis of LUX-lung 3/6: track: advanced NSCLC. J Thorac Oncol 2016;11(10):S202–3.

78. Crinò L, Cappuzzo F, Zatloukal P, et al. Gefitinib versus vinorelbine in chemotherapy-naïve elderly patients with advanced non–small-cell lung cancer (INVITE): a randomized, phase II study. J Clin Oncol 2008;26(26):4253–60.

79. Maemondo M, Minegishi Y, Inoue A, et al. First-line gefitinib in patients aged 75 or older with advanced non–small cell lung cancer harboring epidermal growth factor receptor mutations: NEJ 003 study. J Thorac Oncol 2012;7(9):1417–22.

80. Camidge DR, Bang Y-J, Kwak EL, et al. Activity and safety of crizotinib in patients with ALK-positive non-small-cell lung cancer: updated results from a phase 1 study. Lancet Oncol 2012;13(10):1011–9.

81. Brahmer J, Reckamp KL, Baas P, et al. Nivolumab versus Docetaxel in advanced squamous-cell non–small-cell lung cancer. N Engl J Med 2015;373(2):123–35.

82. Borghaei H, Paz-Ares L, Horn L, et al. Nivolumab versus Docetaxel in advanced nonsquamous non–small-cell lung cancer. N Engl J Med 2015;373(17):1627–39.

83. Herbst RS, Baas P, Kim DW, et al. Pembrolizumab versus docetaxel for previously treated, PD-L1-positive, advanced non-small-cell lung cancer (KEYNOTE-010): a randomised controlled trial. Lancet 2016;387(10027):1540–50.

84. Rittmeyer A, Barlesi F, Waterkamp D, et al. Atezolizumab versus docetaxel in patients with previously treated non-small-cell lung cancer (OAK): a phase 3, open-label, multicentre randomised controlled trial. Lancet 2017;389(10066):255–65.

85. Reck M, Rodriguez-Abreu D, Robinson AG, et al. Pembrolizumab versus chemotherapy for PD-L1-positive non-small cell lung cancer. N Engl J Med 2016; 375(19):1823–33.

86. Antonia SJ, Lopez-Martin JA, Bendell J, et al. Nivolumab alone and nivolumab plus ipilimumab in recurrent small-cell lung cancer (CheckMate 032): a multicentre, open-label, phase 1/2 trial. Lancet Oncol 2016;17(7):883–95.

Sleep in the Elderly
Unanswered Questions

Steven H. Feinsilver, MD[a],*, Adam B. Hernandez, MD[b]

KEYWORDS

- Sleep • Elderly • REM behavior disorder • Insomnia • Sleep apnea

KEY POINTS

- Sleep normally changes with aging, with implications for healthy elderly individuals as well as for those with disease states.
- Less slow wave sleep (deep sleep) is expected, along with more awakenings, and a tendency toward earlier sleep times.
- Rapid eye movement sleep behavior disorder is seen primarily in elderly individuals, in whom it often represents the earliest sign of a chronic and progressive neurologic disease.
- Complaints of difficulty initiating and maintaining sleep (insomnia) become more common with aging.
- Irregular breathing with sleep also becomes more common, with an increased Apnea Hypopnea Index that may not always be clinically important.

Elderly individuals represent the fastest growing segment of the world's population. Sleep problems in elderly individuals are so common that it is difficult to know with certainty what is normal in this group. This is even more difficult in elderly subjects with nearly any chronic medical condition, as the effects on sleep are often significant. In this article, we first briefly review normal sleep, and then 3 common clinical problems in this population: rapid eye movement (REM) behavior disorder, insomnia, and sleep-disordered breathing.

NORMAL SLEEP

Human consciousness can be thought of as having 3 states: wake, non-REM sleep, and REM sleep. Our current system for scoring sleep has changed very little since its first description by Rechshaffen and Kales in 1968.[1] Polysomnography (ie, a

Adapted in part from Hernandez AB, Feinsilver SH. Sleep in the elderly: normal and abnormal. In: Pandi Perumal SR, editor. Synopsis of Sleep Medicine. Waretown (NJ): Apple Academic Press; 2016, with permission.
[a] Hofstra Northwell School of Medicine, Center for Sleep Medicine, Lenox Hill Hospital, 100 East 77th Street, New York, NY, USA; [b] Sleep Disorders Centers of the Mid-Atlantic, 7671 Quarterfield Road, Suite 201, Glen Burnie, MD 21061, USA
* Corresponding author.
E-mail address: sfeinsil@northwell.edu

sleep study) involves at a minimum the recording of electroencephalography (EEG), muscle tone via electromyography (EMG), and eye movements (electrooculography). Respiration is monitored by recording airflow with nasal pressure sensors and thermistors, respiratory effort with measurement of chest and abdominal movement, and oximetry. Electrocardiography is monitored. Leg movements are often recorded using EMG on the anterior tibialis muscle. Additional recordings may be occasionally necessary.

An outline of the characteristics of normal human sleep stages is shown in **Table 1**. EEG during wakefulness is mostly a low-amplitude, high-frequency signal with relatively high muscle tone on EMG. During relaxed quiet wakefulness, alpha activity predominates on the EEG (8–12 Hz), shown in **Fig. 1**. The transition from wake to sleep is characterized by a reduction in EMG amplitude, and the disappearance of alpha activity on the EEG, which is replaced by a low-amplitude mixed-frequency signal. Slow ("rolling") eye movements may be seen. Stage 1 non-REM sleep is light sleep during which the subject can be easily awakened, and is considered transitional to deeper sleep stages. In stage 2, making up approximately half of the total sleep period, characteristic sleep spindles (brief episodes of 12–14-Hz activity lasting at least 0.5 seconds) and K complexes (fast biphasic waves beginning with a sharp upward deflection) are seen. Examples of spindles and K complexes are shown in **Fig. 2**. In stage 3 sleep, slow waves of 0.5-Hz to 2.0-Hz frequency with an amplitude of greater than 75 μV make up at least 20% of the tracing. Examples of slow waves are seen in **Fig. 3**. This is the deepest stage of human sleep.

REM sleep has been said to be as different from non-REM sleep as it is from wakefulness. It was originally termed "paradoxic sleep"; the paradox being that the brain appears active with voluntary muscles being nearly paralyzed. The EEG combines aspects of wakefulness and stage 1 sleep. Striking REMs are seen (**Fig. 4**). There is a decrease in muscle tone on the EMG to the lowest level of the night. Most well-defined dreams are thought to occur in REM sleep. REM is also the time of greatest cardiac and respiratory instability during the sleep period.

WHAT IS NORMAL SLEEP IN HEALTHY ELDERLY INDIVIDUALS?

Defining normal sleep in elderly individuals is problematic. Changes occur in both sleep timing and quality. Two popular assumptions are that older people need less sleep and are more likely to be sleepy during the day. Neither may be true, at least in healthy elderly individuals. It does at least appear to be true that with aging, subjects get less nocturnal sleep.

Insomnia can be defined as difficulty falling asleep, difficulty staying asleep, or the perception of nonrestorative sleep. Some of these complaints may be the norm in

Table 1 Normal sleep		
Stage	**Characteristics**	**Significance**
Wake	Alpha activity	
1	Alpha absent, slow eye movements	Light ("transitional") sleep
2	Spindles, K complexes	Approximately 50% of normal night
3	Slow waves ("delta waves")	Deepest, most restorative sleep
Rapid eye movement	Rapid eye movements, reduced muscle tone	Most dreaming occurs

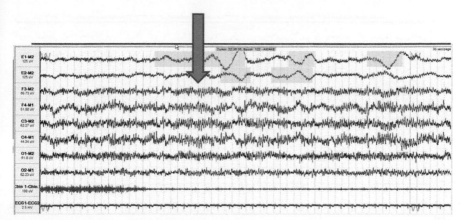

Fig. 1. Wakefulness. This and the following figures are 30-second samples of EEG leads (F: frontal, C: central, O: occipital), eye movements (E), EMG from chin, and electrocardiogram. This tracing shows predominately alpha activity (*arrow*).

elderly individuals. A typical feature of geriatric sleep is a decline in sleep efficiency, defined as the ratio of time asleep to time in bed. This is mostly because of multiple nocturnal awakenings, which are a frequent complaint. An increase in time needed to fall asleep (sleep latency) is a less common chief complaint. In addition to changes with normal aging, disease and medication may cause decreased sleep efficiency. As examples, patients with chronic lung disease may have their sleep disturbed by dyspnea or cough, and patients taking diuretics may wake to urinate.

Age-related changes in polysomnographic parameters have been somewhat inconsistent in the literature. Most studies have shown reductions in total sleep time, sleep efficiency, and slow wave sleep, with an increase in wake after sleep onset. Changes in REM sleep and sleep latency have been less consistent. The Sleep Heart Health Study (2004)[2] found a notable decline in slow wave sleep with aging in its random sample of men, but this was not seen in women. REM sleep declined modestly in both men and women. In contrast, a meta-analysis of 65 studies done by Ohayon and colleagues[3] showed a decline in total sleep time, sleep efficiency, slow wave sleep, and the percentage of REM sleep from young adulthood to elderly subjects

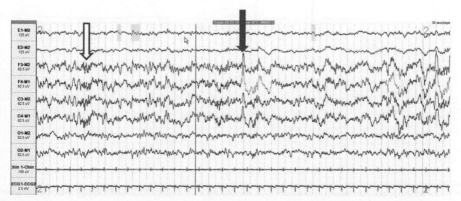

Fig. 2. Stage 2 sleep, showing spindles (*open arrow*) and K complexes (*filled arrow*).

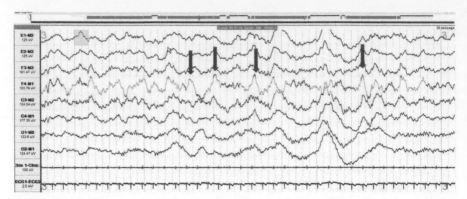

Fig. 3. Stage 3 (slow wave) sleep. Arrows mark several slow waves, also known as delta waves.

in both genders. With advanced age, wake after sleep onset was increased and the percentage of stage 1 and stage 2 sleep was increased. Interestingly, sleep latency was not changed.

A recent study in Brazil sampled 1024 random individuals without significant "mental and physical disturbances" from age 20 to 80.[4] There was a fairly linear increase in wake after sleep onset with aging. Smaller effect sizes were seen for increases in sleep latency, REM latency, and percentages of stage 1 and 2. Total sleep time, sleep efficiency, and slow wave sleep were reduced with aging. The effects were not gender specific.

The reduction in slow wave sleep seen with aging is mostly seen from adulthood to middle age. Normally, most growth hormone production occurs in slow wave sleep. With the reduction in slow wave sleep in aging, there is also a parallel decrease in growth hormone secretion in men, suggesting this does have physiologic significance.[5]

ARE HEALTHY ELDERLY SUBJECTS SLEEPIER?

The significance of changes in sleep in healthy elderly individuals is best assessed by measuring daytime functioning and daytime sleepiness. The most well-validated

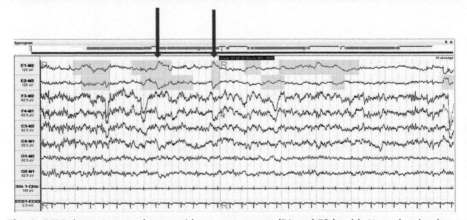

Fig. 4. REM sleep. Arrows show rapid eye movements (E1 and E2 leads). Note that leads are placed so that eye movements appear to have opposite directions.

measure of daytime sleepiness is the multiple sleep latency test (MSLT), although this has been criticized as testing the ability to fall asleep rather than the ability to maintain wakefulness. Earlier studies have suggested that older people are sleepier.[6] However, in a study of 110 healthy subjects, there was an age-related reduction in daytime sleep propensity on the MSLT, despite an increase in wake after sleep onset, reduction in slow wave sleep, and sleep continuity.[7] This somewhat unexpected finding may be due to the time of day MSLT testing is generally performed, as testing ends before the evening hours when older adults may be sleepier than younger adults. A small study of 26 young versus 11 elderly subjects suggested healthy elderly subjects were less sleepy and did better after sleep deprivation than younger subjects.[8]

In the Cardiovascular Health Study, with 4578 adults older than 65, 20% of participants reported being "usually sleepy in the daytime." However, by design, this was not a selected population of elderly subjects; comorbidities were allowed, and sleepiness was more common in those with depression, loud snoring, heart failure, and sedentary lifestyle, among other factors.[9]

Circadian rhythms also change with aging, generally becoming weaker.[10] This likely relates to deterioration of the suprachiasmatic nucleus, with decreased response to external time cues and decreased melatonin secretion. The most important time cue is light exposure. In many elderly subjects, exposure to natural light may be diminished, especially in the institutionalized elderly, and sensitivity may be reduced by reduced visual acuity. Stereotypically, there is a shift toward earlier bedtime and wake time (circadian phase advance). Social pressure to maintain sleep times more typical of the general population may cause many elderly patients to go to bed later than their optimal circadian time, leading to sleep loss.

Many patients will compensate for decreased sleep at night by napping during the day. It is unclear whether this is beneficial. In one study of 455 70-year-old subjects followed for 12 years, survival was significantly reduced in those who reported napping. In fact, napping appeared to be a significant independent predictor of mortality.[11] The investigators could not distinguish voluntary napping from fatigue, and did not recommend abstaining from napping. In another study of 33 healthy subjects between 55 and 85 years old, the opportunity to nap in the midafternoon improved cognitive performance with little effect on subsequent nighttime sleep quality or duration.[12] Most elderly patients complaining of insufficient nocturnal sleep should be encouraged to nap.

As in the rest of the population, those with excessive daytime somnolence need to be evaluated for sleep deprivation, mood disorders, medical illness, or primary sleep disorders.

A summary of changes in sleep in healthy elderly individuals is shown in **Table 2**.

Table 2 Sleep in the healthy elderly	
Parameter	**Characteristic**
Total sleep time (TST)	Reduced
Sleep efficiency (SE)	Reduced
Wake after sleep onset (WASO)	Increased
Rapid eye movement (REM) sleep	Slightly increased
Sleep latency	Increased
REM latency	Probably reduced
Slow wave sleep (SWS)	Reduced
Sleep latency (on Multiple Sleep Latency Test)	Possibly increased

WHAT IS A NORMAL SLEEP SCHEDULE IN ELDERLY INDIVIDUALS?

The habitual bedtime and waketime of an elderly subject frequently tends to be earlier. Attempts to either delay bedtime or stay in bed in the morning to delay wake time may result in sleep restriction, sleepiness, and insomnia (early morning awakening). The delay in bedtime is often sought for social reasons, sometimes in an effort to synchronize with the sleep-wake schedule of a spouse or partner. Sleepiness is usually maximal in the late afternoon and early evening, but may be present to some extent throughout the day,[13] especially if significant sleep restriction is present.

Elderly patients may be retired or partially retired and more able to conform to earlier sleep times. Prevalence of an early sleep and wake schedule increases with age and this may be more common in men.[14–16] Importantly, early morning awakening is a common symptom of depression in elderly individuals,[17] and this diagnosis should be ruled out with care.

Evening bright light therapy (between 7 PM and 9 PM) has been shown to delay circadian phase and reduce awakenings in multiple studies, including one of elderly subjects, although positive results have not been universal.[17–21] Other potential options include chronotherapy (progressive advancement of bed time) and morning melatonin, although neither is a proven therapy.[22,23]

RAPID EYE MOVEMENT SLEEP BEHAVIOR DISORDER

REM sleep behavior disorder (RBD) is characterized by loss of the muscle paralysis seen in normal REM sleep, allowing patients to act out their dreams. This disorder has an increased prevalence in elderly subjects and may coexist with or precede by many years the diagnosis of Parkinson disease (PD) or other neurodegenerative disorders.[24]

Clinical Characteristics

Patients usually present with concerns over dream-enacting behavior (DEB), which may range in manifestation from brief jerking movements and vocalizations to violent thrashing, hitting, kicking, yelling, and/or falling out of bed.[25] Episodes may occur up to several times per week and are more frequent during the latter half of the sleep period. Patients infrequently sleep-walk or leave the bedroom; such behavior is more likely to be related to a non-REM (NREM) parasomnia. DEB may result in injury to the patient (most often due to falling out of bed) or bed partner. Vocalizations may be loud, emotional, and contain language and expletives that may be uncharacteristic of the patient during wakefulness.[26] If patients awaken, they often remember the content of their dreams and the bed partner may be able to correlate this with the specific DEB. Importantly, patients are alert and do not have sustained confusion on awakening, which may aid in distinguishing the disorder from an NREM parasomnia. Symptoms of RBD usually manifest in late adulthood and the diagnosis is often delayed for several years.[24]

RBD may manifest in patients with known neurodegenerative disorders or may predate symptoms and diagnosis by months to decades. Among patients with idiopathic RBD, approximately 40% to 75% will develop PD, multiple system atrophy (MSA), or dementia with Lewy bodies (DLB) in 10 years,[27] and up to 90% at 14 years.[28] The mean time to development of symptoms was 7.5 years in one study.[28] In addition, patients may demonstrate subtle or subclinical signs of impaired motor or cognitive function.[25] Age, family history of dementia, and autonomic and motor symptoms may predict a higher risk of later development of PD, MSA, or DLB.[29]

Epidemiology

RBD is uncommon (overall prevalence 0.5%) but has increased prevalence in elderly individuals (possibly as high as 2%) with a strong male predominance.[25,30–33] RBD is very common in patients with movement disorders, with an estimated prevalence of approximately 50% in PD,[33] 70% to 90% in MSA,[34] and 80% in DLB.[35] RBD also may occur less commonly in a variety of other neurologic disorders, including Alzheimer disease, amyotrophic lateral sclerosis, progressive supranuclear palsy, and Huntington disease.[25,36]

Pathophysiology

RBD may occur in a variety of clinical contexts, including neurodegenerative diseases, narcolepsy,[37] pontine lesions,[38] and medications.[39]

It is possible that most cases of idiopathic RBD may be an early manifestation of preclinical PD, MSA, or DLB.[25]

Medication-associated (toxic) RBD is most commonly related to antidepressants (selective serotonin reuptake inhibitors, tricyclic antidepressants, and monoamine oxidase inhibitors) and may occur in up to 6% of patients using them.[24,25] Of note, medication-associated RBD may predict future development of neurodegenerative disease, although not as strongly as idiopathic RBD.[40]

Diagnosis

Diagnosis of RBD requires DEB, polysomnography (PSG), and the fact that the symptoms are not better explained by another disorder or seizures (International Classification of Sleep Disorders, Third Edition [ICSD-3]).[41] DEB is most often documented during the patient's history but also may be observed during PSG with video. Importantly, obstructive sleep apnea (OSA), which is common in elderly individuals, can mimic RBD (pseudo-RBD) and should be ruled out with PSG.[42] Diagnosis of RBD is summarized in **Box 1**.

Treatment

Treatment is aimed at preventing injury to the patient and/or bed partner. Interventions may include environmental safety precautions and pharmacotherapy. In addition, discontinuation of any potential medications that may be causing or contributing to RBD should be considered.[25]

Sleeping environment interventions may include moving dangerous items out of the bedroom, placing a mattress next to the bed, bed rails or other form of barrier to

---

Box 1
Diagnostic criteria for rapid eye movement sleep behavior disorder (International Classification of Sleep Disorders, Third Edition)

Rapid eye movement (REM) sleep without atonia on electromyography recording

Destructive or injurious behavior (dream-enactment behavior) by history or observed during REM sleep on polysomnography with video

Absence of seizure as cause

Symptoms not better explained by another disorder or substance

From American Academy of Sleep Medicine. International classification of sleep disorders. 3rd edition. Darien (IL): American Academy of Sleep Medicine; 2014. p. 246–53; with permission.

prevent falling out of the bed, barriers placed between the patient and spouse, and/or use of a sleeping bag to restrict movement.[26,43]

For patients in whom environmental interventions are insufficient, pharmacotherapy can be considered. Although randomized controlled trials are lacking, the most evidence-based effective treatment for RBD is the benzodiazepine, clonazepam. Low doses (0.5–2.0 mg) at bedtime have been shown to reduce DEB in most patients.[25,44] Of particular concern in elderly individuals, side effects of clonazepam are not uncommon and include daytime sedation, cognitive impairment, and falls; thus, this agent should be used with caution in this population.[45,46]

Alternatively, melatonin, an over-the-counter agent, may be useful in patients who develop side effects on clonazepam or who are at high risk of side effects. Relatively high doses of melatonin (6–15 mg) have been shown in case series to restore REM atonia and reduce DEB.[47,48] Melatonin may have a more favorable side-effect profile in elderly individuals, but there is less experience treating RBD with this drug.[49] A variety of other medications have been used in the treatment of RBD, but overall evidence for use of these agents is scant and/or conflicting.[43,46,50]

Finally, patients with idiopathic RBD should be informed of the risk of future development of neurologic disease and appropriate counseling and/or neurology referral might be offered.[51]

WHAT IS INSOMNIA, AND WHEN SHOULD IT BE TREATED IN ELDERLY INDIVIDUALS?

Insomnia is a common complaint in the general population, but it is especially prevalent in elderly individuals, and treatment poses specific challenges in this population. In particular, elderly individuals suffer from higher rates of comorbid disease and may be at higher risk of adverse effects of hypnotic medications.

Clinical Characteristics

Insomnia is defined as difficulty initiating or maintaining sleep in combination with daytime symptoms. It is important to differentiate this from simply short sleep time, which may or may not be problematic. Although previous classifications have differentiated primary and comorbid insomnia and subclassified primary insomnias (ie, psychophysiological, idiopathic, paradoxic), the recent ICSD-3 has grouped most of these previous classifications under the term "chronic insomnia."[41] Insomnia is associated with poorer physical function, cognitive decline, lower quality of life, depression, falls, and mortality, although it is often uncertain whether this is a cause or effect.[52–57]

Epidemiology

Insomnia increases in prevalence with age and may affect up to one-third of older adults.[58,59] In older adults, data from the Sleep Heart Health Study showed a higher rate of subjective sleep complaints in women, whereas men had greater abnormalities in sleep architecture.[59] In addition, older age may be a risk factor for persistence of symptoms.[60] Insomnia is more common in older adults with higher rates of chronic medical and psychiatric disease.[61]

Pathophysiology

Certain etiologic factors are specific to or particularly important in elderly individuals. Older adults have a higher rate of chronic, comorbid diseases (eg, depression, memory impairment, chronic pain, heart disease) and poor overall health, which correlates with an increased risk of insomnia.[61–63] Medication side effects may be a factor in insomnia.[64] Psychosocial factors common to elderly individuals also may play a role. Both lower levels of physical activity and caregiver status have been identified as risk factors for insomnia in this population.[63,65,66] In a recent study, self-reported poor sleep in older subjects was more common in African American individuals and those with fewer years of education.[67]

Age-related circadian factors noted previously may lead to irregularity in sleep schedule and early morning awakening.[68]

Diagnosis

Insomnia is a clinical diagnosis based on reported difficulty initiating or maintaining sleep in combination with daytime complaints and in the setting of adequate sleep opportunity and environment (ICSD-3).[41]

Treatment

Treatment options include behavioral therapies, pharmacotherapy, and psychosocial interventions.

Behavioral treatments (including cognitive behavioral therapy for insomnia) have proven effective for treating insomnia in older adults in randomized controlled trials.[69–71] Compared with hypnotic medications, behavioral therapies demonstrate similar (or better) short-term efficacy and improved long-term efficacy, and are considered the first-line approach in consensus guidelines.[64,72,73]

As pharmacotherapy options, nonbenzodiazepine benzodiazepine receptor agonists such as zaleplon and zopiclone and low-dose doxepin have been shown to be effective at improving sleep in elderly individuals in randomized trials.[74–77] In addition, ramelteon, a melatonin receptor agonist, and prolonged release melatonin have been specifically studied in elderly individuals, with modest benefit and minimal adverse effects.[78–80]

Multiple studies appear to show an increased risk of adverse events in elderly patients taking hypnotics for treatment of insomnia. Both benzodiazepines and nonbenzodiazepine hypnotics are associated with an increased risk of hip fractures in elderly individuals,[81–84] although one study correlated falls with sleep disturbance and not with hypnotic use.[55] A large meta-analysis showed a significantly increased risk of adverse cognitive events, adverse psychomotor events, and daytime fatigue in older adults taking hypnotics for insomnia.[85] The American Geriatrics Society has released recommendations to avoid the use of benzodiazepine medications for insomnia in elderly individuals (and to avoid using other hypnotics for more than 90 days) due to the risk of adverse effects.[86] If expertise is available, cognitive behavioral therapy is the preferred technique when attempting to taper older patients off chronic hypnotic therapy.[87]

Frequent physical activity may protect against insomnia in elderly individuals.[88–91] A recent randomized trial of a cognitive intervention showed improvements in sleep quality in older adults.[92] In sum, the evidence suggests that structured exercise and possibly social activities may be beneficial in older patients with insomnia. In light of the minimal risk incurred by these interventions and potential other benefits, these options should be considered in addition to behavioral and possibly pharmacologic therapies. As always, sleep may be optimized by light exposure in the morning and darkness in the evening, conditions not always easy to maintain in the institutionalized elderly. Issues of insomnia in elderly individuals are summarized in **Box 2**.

DOES SLEEP-DISORDERED BREATHING GET WORSE WITH AGING?

It has been suggested that in older adults sleep apnea is a different disorder with a distinct phenotype.[93,94] With aging, there is an increased tendency for upper airway

> **Box 2**
> **Issues in insomnia in elderly individuals**
>
> Higher prevalence than in general population
>
> High prevalence of comorbid chronic medical or psychiatric disease
>
> Increased risk of side effects from hypnotic medications
>
> Advanced sleep-wake phase disorder is common
>
> Decreased exposure to natural light, exercise, and social interactions during the day
>
> Normal changes with aging may be misperceived as illness

collapse with lengthening of the soft palate and increased upper airway fat.[95] Some, but not all, studies show increased airway collapsibility with aging,[96] although there also may be increased upper airway size.[97,98] It appears the increase in OSA with aging is primarily because of changes in the anatomy and physiology of the upper airway.[94]

Clinical Characteristics and Epidemiology

The prevalence of OSA clearly increases with age. Sleep apnea is generally quantified by the number of times per hour that patients stop or reduce their breathing, the Apnea Hypopnea Index (AHI). In the Sleep Heart Health Study, the prevalence of sleep apnea in the general population was 1.7 times higher in those older than 60 compared with 40-year-old to 60-year-old adults.[99] Nineteen percent of those between 60 and 69, and 21% of those 70 to 79 had an AHI greater than or equal to 15. In a study of community-dwelling adults 62 to 91 years old, nearly one-third had an AHI of 15 or more.[100] The prevalence of sleep apnea increases in patients who are generally less healthy, and is higher in institutionalized compared with independently living elderly.[101]

Sleep apnea may present differently in elderly individuals. In the Sleep Heart Health Study, it was found that elderly subjects were much less likely to report witnessed apneas.[99] The male predominance of OSA appears to disappear after approximately age 50, probably because of the effects of menopause.[102] Surprisingly, one community study suggests that the effects of obesity on the prevalence of sleep apnea may be negligible in those at or beyond 60 years of age.[103] In an observational study of 389 consecutive patients with sleep apnea, patients 65 years or older did not differ significantly in terms of disease severity, PSG findings, or the therapeutic implications of their diagnostic study when compared with younger patients.[104]

At least when severe, untreated sleep apnea is clearly associated with increased mortality and multiple morbidities. However, these associations are less well established in elderly individuals. In a prospective cohort study following 6441 adults for an average of 8 years, untreated severe sleep apnea, defined as an AHI greater than 30, was associated with increased mortality compared with those with an AHI less than 5.[105] However, in the subgroup of 110 adults older than 70 years, untreated severe sleep apnea was not associated with increased mortality (relative risk 1.27, 95% confidence interval [CI] 0.86–1.86 among men; relative risk 1.14, 95% CI 0.65–2.01 among women).

Untreated sleep apnea has been linked to increased risk for stroke.[106] In a 6-year follow-up of a cohort of 400 adults aged 72 to 100, patients with untreated severe sleep apnea had an increased risk of developing and ischemic stroke compared with those without apnea (adjusted hazard ratio 2.52, 95% CI 1.04–6.01).[107]

Dementia and milder forms of cognitive impairment are of extreme importance in older adults. Several observational studies have found an association between sleep apnea and cognitive defects. In one prospective study, 298 women with a mean age of 82 years were followed for 4 years with cognitive testing.[108] Women with sleep apnea, as defined as AHI greater than or equal to 15, were more likely to develop mild cognitive defects or dementia compared with women without sleep apnea (45 vs 31%, adjusted odds ratio 1.85, 95% CI 1.11–3.08).

Untreated sleep apnea is also associated with hypertension. Data from the Sleep Heart Health Study show a closer association with time spent below 90% oxygen saturation and hypertension in those older than 65 years than in younger subjects.[109] The AHI did not predict hypertension. Other studies that have used the AHI alone have shown a reduced association between sleep apnea and systemic hypertension with increasing age.[110,111]

In a prospective cohort of the Sleep Heart Health Study of 4422 adults followed for almost 9 years, untreated severe sleep apnea (AHI greater than or equal to 30) was associated with an increased risk of coronary artery disease in men between 40 and 70 years of age. This effect was not seen in older men or in women.[112] Other studies have had too few events to confirm this association in elderly individuals.[105] Heart failure also may be associated with untreated severe sleep apnea in both older and younger men, but the data from the previously cited study shows only a trend (adjusted hazard ratio 1.58, 95% CI 0.93–2.66).[112]

There is some reason to believe that the effects of sleep apnea might be reduced in older adults; in a study in rats, older animals show less evidence of oxidative stress than younger animals in response to repetitive airway obstruction.[113] In general, however, it is likely that the consequences of OSA are similar in elderly individuals but more difficult to prove because of comorbid illnesses.

Diagnosis

As in younger adults, the most common symptoms of sleep apnea are excessive daytime sleepiness and snoring. Cognitive deficits and nocturia may be more frequent presentations of sleep apnea in elderly individuals, and may be easily attributed to other etiologies in this age group. Sleepiness and attention problems may be more difficult to recognize in patients who are not working or otherwise required to keep a consistent schedule. As the normal AHI may be different in elderly individuals, it remains controversial at what point elderly patients should be treated, particularly in those who do not have significant symptoms or comorbidities. See **Box 3** for a summary of issues regarding sleep apnea in elderly individuals.

Box 3
Obstructive sleep apnea in elderly individuals

High prevalence of at least mild sleep-disordered breathing.

Comorbid pulmonary or cardiac disease more common

More frequent nighttime awakenings may make use of continuous positive airway pressure more difficult

Reduction in cardiovascular and cerebrovascular risk with treatment is likely

Increasing evidence that treatment may reduce cognitive decline

WHO SHOULD BE TREATED FOR SLEEP APNEA?

The prevalence of some measurable apnea in elderly individuals is so great that it becomes difficult to define when this is a disease that needs to be treated. Treatment with positive airway pressure remains the most important modality for sleep apnea, but may be more difficult in older adults. Older adults experience more nocturnal awakenings, and may have more difficulty achieving a good mask fit, especially if they are edentulous. An oral appliance may be useful for patients with mild disease, but this may be a less satisfactory option, as it generally requires adequate dentition. Elderly patients may be poor candidates for a surgical approach to treatment.

As always, avoiding alcohol and any sedative medications is important if possible, as their use can decrease respiratory drive, worsen upper airway dysfunction during sleep, and severely worsen sleep apnea. Older patients may be more sensitive to these effects.

Data on treatment outcomes are limited. In a recent multicenter trial including 278 adults 65 years or older with newly diagnosed sleep apnea, patients receiving continuous positive airway pressure (CPAP) plus best supportive care had improvement in daytime sleepiness compared with best supportive care alone.[114] Benefits of CPAP were present at 3-month and 12-month time points and correlated with greater CPAP usage. Efficacy may have been limited by a median nightly CPAP usage of only 2 hours despite a high self-reported CPAP adherence rate.

A prospective study of 939 patients 65 or older showed reduced cardiovascular mortality in patients with an AHI greater than or equal to 30 who used CPAP for at least 4 hours a night.[115] A small study has shown improved outcome in patients with stroke and sleep apnea treated with CPAP,[116] and there has been a great deal of interest in the possibility that sleep apnea diagnosis and treatment may aid both stroke prevention and therapy.

There has been some recent evidence that treating sleep apnea may decrease cognitive decline in patients with Alzheimer disease; in a recent study of 23 patients with severe apnea (AHI ≥30), decline in mini mental status examination was slower in those treated with CPAP.[117] A recent study by Osorio and colleagues[118] from the Alzheimer's Disease Neuroimaging Initiative showed that the presence of sleep apnea was associated with an earlier age of cognitive decline that was delayed by treatment with CPAP.

SUMMARY

Some features of sleep even in the completely healthy elderly individuals make it difficult to know when normal aging becomes disease. Nocturnal sleep quality is reduced by most measures, and napping may be appropriate. Advanced sleep phase may be part of normal aging. RBD can be dangerous, and can generally be controlled with medication, but may be the first manifestation of a neurodegenerative disease. Insomnia is highly prevalent, and generally should be treated behaviorally. The observation of sleep apnea is common in elderly individuals, but may not always indicate disease requiring treatment. It is hoped that more data about outcomes will provide further proof that treatment of sleep disorders can significantly improve quality of life, morbidity, and mortality in the expanding aging population.

REFERENCES

1. Rechtschaffen A, Kales A. A manual of standardized terminology, techniques and scoring system for sleep stages of human subjects. Los Angeles (CA): UCLA Brain Information Service/Brain Research Institute; 1968.

2. Redline S, Kirchner HL, Quan SF, et al. The effects of age, sex, ethnicity, and sleep disordered breathing on sleep architecture. Arch Intern Med 2004;164: 406–18.

3. Ohayon MM, Carskadon MA, Guilleminault C, et al. Meta-analysis of quantitative sleep parameters from childhood to old age in healthy individuals: developing normative sleep values across the human lifespans. Sleep 2004;27:1255–73.

4. Moraes W, Piovezan R, Poyares D, et al. Effects of aging on sleep structure through adulthood: a population-based study. Sleep Med 2014;15:401–9.

5. Van Cauter E, Leproult R, Plat L. Age-related changes in slow wave sleep and REM sleep and relationship with growth hormone and cortisol levels in healthy men. JAMA 2000;284:861–8.

6. Carskadon MA, Van den Hoed J, Dement WC. Insomnia and sleep disturbances in the aged. Sleep and daytime sleepiness in the elderly. J Geriatr Psychiatry 1980;13:135–51.

7. Dijk D-J, Groeger JA, Stanley N, et al. Age-related reduction in daytime sleep propensity and nocturnal slow wave sleep. Sleep 2010;33:211–23.

8. Duffy JF, Wilson HJ, Wang W, et al. Healthy older adults better tolerate sleep deprivation than young adults. J Am Geriatr Soc 2009;57:1245–51.

9. Whitney CW, Enright PL, Newman AB, et al. Correlates of daytime sleepiness in 4578 elderly persons: the Cardiovascular Health Study. Sleep 1998;21:27–36.

10. Pandi-Perumal SR, Spence DW, Sharma VK. Aging and circadian rhythms: general trends. In: Pandi-Perumal SR, Monti JM, Monjan AA, editors. Principles and practice of geriatric sleep medicine. Cambridge (UK): Cambridge University Press; 2010. p. 3–11.

11. Bursztyn M, Stessman J. The siesta and mortality: twelve years of prospective observations in 70-year-olds. Sleep 2005;28:345–57.

12. Campbell SS, Murphy PJ, Stauble TN. Effects of a nap on nighttime sleep and waking function in older subjects. J Am Geriatr Soc 2005;53:48–53.

13. Ando K, Kripke DF, Ancoli-Israel S. Delayed and advanced sleep phase symptoms. Isr J Psychiatry Relat Sci 2002;39(1):11–8.

14. Schrader H, Bovim G, Sand T. The prevalence of delayed and advanced sleep phase syndromes. J Sleep Res 1993;2(1):51–5.

15. Paine SJ, Fink J, Gander PH, et al. Identifying advanced and delayed sleep phase disorders in the general population: a national survey of New Zealand adults. Chronobiol Int 2014;31(5):627–36.

16. Carrier J, Monk TH, Buysse DJ, et al. Sleep and morningness-eveningness in the 'middle' years of life (20-59 y). J Sleep Res 1997;6(4):230–7.

17. Lack L, Wright H, Kemp K, et al. The treatment of early-morning awakening insomnia with 2 evenings of bright light. Sleep 2005;28(5):616–23.

18. Suhner AG, Murphy PJ, Campbell SS. Failure of timed bright light exposure to alleviate age-related sleep maintenance insomnia. J Am Geriatr Soc 2002; 50(4):617–23.

19. Campbell SS, Dawson D, Anderson MW. Alleviation of sleep maintenance insomnia with timed exposure to bright light. J Am Geriatr Soc 1993;41(8): 829–36.

20. Lack L, Wright H. The effect of evening bright light in delaying the circadian rhythms and lengthening the sleep of early morning awakening insomniacs. Sleep 1993;16(5):436–43.

21. Pallesen S, Nordhus IH, Skelton SH, et al. Bright light treatment has limited effect in subjects over 55 years with mild early morning awakening. Percept Mot Skills 2005;101(3):759–70.

22. Moldofsky H, Musisi S, Phillipson EA. Treatment of a case of advanced sleep phase syndrome by phase advance chronotherapy. Sleep 1986;9(1):61–5.

23. Zee PC. Melantonin for the treatment of advanced sleep phase disorder. Sleep 2008;31(7):923 [author reply: 925].

24. Olson EJ, Boeve BF, Silber MH. Rapid eye movement sleep behaviour disorder: demographic, clinical and laboratory findings in 93 cases. Brain 2000;123(Pt 2): 331–9.

25. Boeve BF. REM sleep behavior disorder: updated review of the core features, the REM sleep behavior disorder-neurodegenerative disease association, evolving concepts, controversies, and future directions. Ann N Y Acad Sci 2010;1184:15–54.

26. Sasai T, Inoue Y, Matsuura M. Do patients with rapid eye movement sleep behavior disorder have a disease-specific personality? Parkinsonism Relat Disord 2012;18(5):616–8.

27. Postuma RB, Gagnon JF, Vendette M, et al. Quantifying the risk of neurodegenerative disease in idiopathic REM sleep behavior disorder. Neurology 2009; 72(15):1296–300.

28. Iranzo A, Fernández-Arcos A, Tolosa E, et al. Neurodegenerative disorder risk in idiopathic REM sleep behavior disorder: study in 174 patients. PLoS One 2014; 9(2):e89741.

29. Postuma RB, Iranzo A, Hogl B, et al. Risk factors for neurodegeneration in idiopathic rapid eye movement sleep behavior disorder: a multicenter study. Ann Neurol 2015;77(5):830–9.

30. Kang SH, Yoon IY, Lee SD, et al. REM sleep behavior disorder in the Korean elderly population: prevalence and clinical characteristics. Sleep 2013;36(8): 1147–52.

31. Bodkin CL, Schenck CH. Rapid eye movement sleep behavior disorder in women: relevance to general and specialty medical practice. J Womens Health (Larchmt) 2009;18(12):1955–63.

32. Ohayon MM, Caulet M, Priest RG. Violent behavior during sleep. J Clin Psychiatry 1997;58(8):369–76 [quiz: 377].

33. Poryazova R, Oberholzer M, Baumann CR, et al. REM sleep behavior disorder in Parkinson's disease: a questionnaire-based survey. J Clin Sleep Med 2013;9(1): 55-9A.

34. Plazzi G, Corsini R, Provini F, et al. REM sleep behavior disorders in multiple system atrophy. Neurology 1997;48(4):1094–7.

35. Boeve BF, Silber MH, Ferman TJ. REM sleep behavior disorder in Parkinson's disease and dementia with Lewy bodies. J Geriatr Psychiatry Neurol 2004; 17(3):146–57.

36. Wang P, Wing YK, Xing J, et al. Rapid eye movement sleep behavior disorder in patients with probable Alzheimer's disease. Aging Clin Exp Res 2015;28(5): 951–7.

37. Dauvilliers Y, Jennum P, Plazzi G. Rapid eye movement sleep behavior disorder and rapid eye movement sleep without atonia in narcolepsy. Sleep Med 2013; 14(8):775–81.

38. Jianhua C, Xiuqin L, Quancai C, et al. Rapid eye movement sleep behavior disorder in a patient with brainstem lymphoma. Intern Med 2013;52(5):617–21.

39. Teman PT, Tippmann-Peikert M, Silber MH, et al. Idiopathic rapid-eye-movement sleep disorder: associations with antidepressants, psychiatric diagnoses, and other factors, in relation to age of onset. Sleep Med 2009;10(1):60–5.

40. Postuma RB, Gagnon JF, Tuineaig M, et al. Antidepressants and REM sleep behavior disorder: isolated side effect or neurodegenerative signal? Sleep 2013;36(11):1579–85.
41. American Academy of Sleep Medicine. International classification of sleep disorders. 3rd edition. Darien (IL): American Academy of Sleep Medicine; 2014.
42. Iranzo A, Santamaria J. Severe obstructive sleep apnea/hypopnea mimicking REM sleep behavior disorder. Sleep 2005;28(2):203–6.
43. Devnani P, Fernandes R. Management of REM sleep behavior disorder: an evidence based review. Ann Indian Acad Neurol 2015;18(1):1–5.
44. Schenck CH, Hurwitz TD, Mahowald MW. Symposium: normal and abnormal REM sleep regulation: REM sleep behaviour disorder: an update on a series of 96 patients and a review of the world literature. J Sleep Res 1993;2(4):224–31.
45. Gagnon JF, Postuma RB, Montplaisir J. Update on the pharmacology of REM sleep behavior disorder. Neurology 2006;67(5):742–7.
46. Anderson KN, Shneerson JM. Drug treatment of REM sleep behavior disorder: the use of drug therapies other than clonazepam. J Clin Sleep Med 2009;5(3):235–9.
47. Boeve BF, Silber MH, Ferman TJ. Melatonin for treatment of REM sleep behavior disorder in neurologic disorders: results in 14 patients. Sleep Med 2003;4(4):281–4.
48. Kunz D, Mahlberg R. A two-part, double-blind, placebo-controlled trial of exogenous melatonin in REM sleep behaviour disorder. J Sleep Res 2010;19(4):591–6.
49. McCarter SJ, Boswell CL, St Louis EK, et al. Treatment outcomes in REM sleep behavior disorder. Sleep Med 2013;14(3):237–42.
50. Trotti LM. REM sleep behaviour disorder in older individuals: epidemiology, pathophysiology and management. Drugs Aging 2010;27(6):457–70.
51. Vertrees S, Greenough GP. Ethical considerations in REM sleep behavior disorder. Continuum (Minneap Minn) 2013;19(1 Sleep Disorders):199–203.
52. Dam TT, Ewing S, Ancoli-Israel S, et al. Association between sleep and physical function in older men: the osteoporotic fractures in men sleep study. J Am Geriatr Soc 2008;56(9):1665–73.
53. Tworoger SS, Lee S, Schernhammer ES, et al. The association of self-reported sleep duration, difficulty sleeping, and snoring with cognitive function in older women. Alzheimer Dis Assoc Disord 2006;20(1):41–8.
54. Cricco M, Simonsick EM, Foley DJ. The impact of insomnia on cognitive functioning in older adults. J Am Geriatr Soc 2001;49(9):1185–9.
55. Avidan AY, Fries BE, James ML, et al. Insomnia and hypnotic use, recorded in the minimum data set, as predictors of falls and hip fractures in Michigan nursing homes. J Am Geriatr Soc 2005;53(6):955–62.
56. Stone KL, Ewing SK, Ancoli-Israel S, et al. Self-reported sleep and nap habits and risk of mortality in a large cohort of older women. J Am Geriatr Soc 2009;57(4):604–11.
57. Jaussent I, Bouyer J, Ancelin ML, et al. Insomnia and daytime sleepiness are risk factors for depressive symptoms in the elderly. Sleep 2011;34(8):1103–10.
58. Foley DJ, Monjan AA, Brown SL, et al. Sleep complaints among elderly persons: an epidemiologic study of three communities. Sleep 1995;18(6):425–32.
59. Unruh ML, Redline S, An MW, et al. Subjective and objective sleep quality and aging in the sleep heart health study. J Am Geriatr Soc 2008;56(7):1218–27.
60. Morphy H, Dunn KM, Lewis M, et al. Epidemiology of insomnia: a longitudinal study in a UK population. Sleep 2007;30(3):274–80.

61. Vitiello MV, Moe KE, Prinz PN. Sleep complaints cosegregate with illness in older adults: clinical research informed by and informing epidemiological studies of sleep. J Psychosom Res 2002;53(1):555–9.
62. Foley D, Ancoli-Israel S, Britz P, et al. Sleep disturbances and chronic disease in older adults: results of the 2003 National Sleep Foundation Sleep in America Survey. J Psychosom Res 2004;56(5):497–502.
63. Morgan K. Daytime activity and risk factors for late-life insomnia. J Sleep Res 2003;12(3):231–8.
64. Bloom HG, Ahmed I, Alessi CA, et al. Evidence-based recommendations for the assessment and management of sleep disorders in older persons. J Am Geriatr Soc 2009;57(5):761–89.
65. Castro CM, Lee KA, Bliwise DL, et al. Sleep patterns and sleep-related factors between caregiving and non-caregiving women. Behav Sleep Med 2009;7(3):164–79.
66. Wilcox S, King AC. Sleep complaints in older women who are family caregivers. J Gerontol B Psychol Sci Soc Sci 1999;54(3):P189–98.
67. Turner AD, Lim AS, Leurgans SE, et al. Self-reported sleep in older African Americans and white Americans. Ethn Dis 2016;26(4):521–8.
68. Czeisler CA, Dumont M, Duffy JF, et al. Association of sleep-wake habits in older people with changes in output of circadian pacemaker. Lancet 1992;340(8825):933–6.
69. Epstein DR, Sidani S, Bootzin RR, et al. Dismantling multicomponent behavioral treatment for insomnia in older adults: a randomized controlled trial. Sleep 2012;35(6):797–805.
70. Mitchell MD, Gehrman P, Perlis M, et al. Comparative effectiveness of cognitive behavioral therapy for insomnia: a systematic review. BMC Fam Pract 2012;13:40.
71. Irwin MR, Cole JC, Nicassio PM. Comparative meta-analysis of behavioral interventions for insomnia and their efficacy in middle-aged adults and in older adults 55+ years of age. Health Psychol 2006;25(1):3–14.
72. Morin CM, Colecchi C, Stone J, et al. Behavioral and pharmacological therapies for late-life insomnia: a randomized controlled trial. JAMA 1999;281(11):991–9.
73. Sivertsen B, Omvik S, Pallesen S, et al. Cognitive behavioral therapy vs zopiclone for treatment of chronic primary insomnia in older adults: a randomized controlled trial. JAMA 2006;295(24):2851–8.
74. Ancoli-Israel S, Walsh JK, Mangano RM, et al. Zaleplon, a novel nonbenzodiazepine hypnotic, effectively treats insomnia in elderly patients without causing rebound effects. Prim Care Companion J Clin Psychiatry 1999;1(4):114–20.
75. Scharf M, Erman M, Rosenberg R, et al. A 2-week efficacy and safety study of eszopiclone in elderly patients with primary insomnia. Sleep 2005;28(6):720–7.
76. Scharf M, Rogowski R, Hull S, et al. Efficacy and safety of doxepin 1 mg, 3 mg, and 6 mg in elderly patients with primary insomnia: a randomized, double-blind, placebo-controlled crossover study. J Clin Psychiatry 2008;69(10):1557–64.
77. Krystal AD, Durrence HH, Scharf M, et al. Efficacy and safety of doxepin 1 mg and 3 mg in a 12-week sleep laboratory and outpatient trial of elderly subjects with chronic primary insomnia. Sleep 2010;33(11):1553–61.
78. Roth T, Seiden D, Wang-Weigand S, et al. A 2-night, 3-period, crossover study of ramelteon's efficacy and safety in older adults with chronic insomnia. Curr Med Res Opin 2007;23(5):1005–14.
79. Lemoine P, Nir T, Laudon M, et al. Prolonged-release melatonin improves sleep quality and morning alertness in insomnia patients aged 55 years and older and has no withdrawal effects. J Sleep Res 2007;16(4):372–80.

80. Wade AG, Ford I, Crawford G, et al. Efficacy of prolonged release melatonin in insomnia patients aged 55-80 years: quality of sleep and next-day alertness outcomes. Curr Med Res Opin 2007;23(10):2597–605.

81. Wang PS, Bohn RL, Glynn RJ, et al. Zolpidem use and hip fractures in older people. J Am Geriatr Soc 2001;49(12):1685–90.

82. Cumming RG, Le Couteur DG. Benzodiazepines and risk of hip fractures in older people: a review of the evidence. CNS Drugs 2003;17(11):825–37.

83. Berry SD, Lee Y, Cai S, et al. Nonbenzodiazepine sleep medication use and hip fractures in nursing home residents. JAMA Intern Med 2013;173(9):754–61.

84. Kang DY, Park S, Rhee CW, et al. Zolpidem use and risk of fracture in elderly insomnia patients. J Prev Med Public Health 2012;45(4):219–26.

85. Glass J, Lanctôt KL, Herrmann N, et al. Sedative hypnotics in older people with insomnia: meta-analysis of risks and benefits. BMJ 2005;331(7526):1169.

86. American Geriatrics Society 2012 Beers Criteria Update Expert Panel. American Geriatrics Society updated Beers Criteria for potentially inappropriate medication use in older adults. J Am Geriatr Soc 2012;60(4):616–31.

87. Morin CM, Bastien C, Guay B, et al. Randomized clinical trial of supervised tapering and cognitive behavior therapy to facilitate benzodiazepine discontinuation in older adults with chronic insomnia. Am J Psychiatry 2004;161(2): 332–42.

88. Inoue S, Yorifuji T, Sugiyama M, et al. Does habitual physical activity prevent insomnia? A cross-sectional and longitudinal study of elderly Japanese. J Aging Phys Act 2013;21(2):119–39.

89. Benloucif S, Orbeta L, Ortiz R, et al. Morning or evening activity improves neuropsychological performance and subjective sleep quality in older adults. Sleep 2004;27(8):1542–51.

90. Naylor E, Penev PD, Orbeta L, et al. Daily social and physical activity increases slow-wave sleep and daytime neuropsychological performance in the elderly. Sleep 2000;23(1):87–95.

91. King AC, Oman RF, Brassington GS, et al. Moderate-intensity exercise and self-rated quality of sleep in older adults. A randomized controlled trial. JAMA 1997; 277(1):32–7.

92. Haimov I, Shatil E. Cognitive training improves sleep quality and cognitive function among older adults with insomnia. PLoS One 2013;8(4):e61390.

93. Launois SH, Pepin J-L, Levy P. Sleep apnea in the elderly: a specific entity? Sleep Med Rev 2007;11:87–97.

94. Edwards BE, Wellman A, Sands SA, et al. Obstructive sleep apnea in older adults is a distinctly different physiological phenotype. Sleep 2014;37(7): 1227–36.

95. Malhotra A, Huang Y, Fogel R, et al. Aging influences on pharyngeal anatomy and physiology: the predisposition to pharyngeal collapse. Am J Med 2006; 119:e9–14.

96. Eikermann M, Jordann AS, Chamberlin NL, et al. The influence of aging on pharyngeal collapsibility during sleep. Chest 2007;131:1702–9.

97. Mayer P, Pepin JL, Bettega G, et al. Relationship between body mass index, age and upper airway measurements in snorers and sleep apnoea patients. Eur Respir J 1996;9:1801–9.

98. Burger CD, Stanson AW, Sheedy PF II, et al. Fast-computed tomography evaluation of age-related changes in upper airway structure and function in normal men. Am Rev Respir Dis 1992;145:846–52.

99. Young T, Shahar E, Nieto FJ, et al. Predictors of sleep disordered breathing in community dwelling adults: the Sleep Heart Health Study. Arch Intern Med 2002;162:893.
100. Endeshaw Y. Clinical characteristics of obstructive sleep apnea in community-dwelling older adults. J Am Geriatr Soc 2006;54:1740–4.
101. Ancoli-Israel S. Epidemiology of sleep disorders. Clin Geriatr Med 1989;5:347.
102. Young T, Finn L, Austin D, et al. Menopausal status and sleep-disordered breathing in the Wisconsin sleep cohort study. Am J Respir Crit Care Med 2003;167:1181–5.
103. Tishler PV, Larkin EK, Schluchter MD, et al. Incidence of sleep-disordered breathing in an urban adult population. JAMA 2003;289:2230–7.
104. Levy P, Pepin JL, Malauzat D, et al. Is sleep apnea syndrome in the elderly a specific entity? Sleep 1996;19:S29.
105. Punjabi NM, Caffo BS, Goodwin JL, et al. Sleep disordered breathing and mortality: a prospective cohort study. PLoS Med 2009;6:e1000132.
106. Yaggi HK, Concato J, Kernan WN, et al. Obstructive sleep apnea as a risk factor for stroke and death. N Engl J Med 2005;353:2034–41.
107. Munoz R, Duran-Cantolla J, Martinez-Vila E, et al. Severe sleep apnea and risk of ischemic stroke in the elderly. Stroke 2006;37:2317.
108. Yaffe K, Laffan AM, Harrison SL, et al. Sleep disordered breathing, hypoxia, and risk of mild cognitive impairment and dementia in older women. JAMA 2011; 306:613.
109. Nieto FJ, Young TB, Lind BK, et al. Association of sleep disordered breathing, sleep apnea, and hypertension in a large community-based study. Sleep Heart Health Study. JAMA 2000;283:1829.
110. Bixler EO, Vgontzas AN, Lin HM, et al. Association of hypertension and sleep disordered breathing. Arch Intern Med 2000;160:2289.
111. Grote L, Ploch T, Heitmann J, et al. Sleep-related breathing disorder is an independent risk factor for systemic hypertension. Am J Respir Crit Care Med 1999; 160:1875.
112. Gottlieb DJ, Yenokyan G, Newman AB, et al. Prospective study of obstructive sleep apnea and incident coronary heart disease and heart failure: the Sleep Heart Health Study. Circulation 2010;122:352.
113. Dalmases M, Torres M, Marquez-Kisinousky L, et al. Brain tissue hypoxia and oxidative stress induced by obstructive apneas is different in young and aged rats. Sleep 2014;37:1249.
114. McMillan A, Bratton DJ, Faria R, et al. Continuous positive airway pressure in older people with obstructive sleep apnoea syndrome (PREDICT): a 12 month multicentre, randomised trial. Lancet Respir Med 2014;2:804.
115. Martinez-Garcia MA, Campos-Rodriquez F, Catalan-Serra P, et al. Cardiovascular mortality in obstructive sleep apnea in the elderly: role of long-term continuous positive airway pressure treatment: a prospective observational study. Am J Respir Crit Care Med 2012;186:909–16.
116. Ryan CM, Bayley M, Green R, et al. Influence of CPAP on outcomes of rehabilitation in stroke patients with OSA. Stroke 2011;42:1062–7.
117. Troussiere AC, Charley CM, Salleron J, et al. Treatment of sleep apnoea syndrome decreases cognitive decline in patients with Alzheimer's disease. J Neurol Neurosurg Psychiatr 2014;85(12):1405–8.
118. Osorio RS, Gumb T, Pirraglia MA, et al. Sleep-disordered breathing advances cognitive decline in the elderly. Neurology 2015;84:1964–71.

Comorbidities of Lung Disease in the Elderly

Nicola Scichilone, MD, PhD

KEYWORDS

- Comorbidity • Senile lung • Aging • Asthma
- Chronic obstructive pulmonary disease • Idiopathic lung fibrosis

KEY POINTS

- Chronic respiratory diseases in older populations are often accompanied by comorbid conditions.
- Comorbidities can affect the manifestations and severity of the underlying lung disease.
- Comorbidities should be taken into account when managing underlying lung disease and should be treated directly.
- A comprehensive and multidimensional approach is encouraged in older populations suffering from chronic respiratory diseases.

INTRODUCTION

Respiratory diseases in elderly individuals are often accompanied by nonrespiratory pathologic conditions. The latter are usually the consequence of the respiratory disease or share the same risk factors (ie, smoking exposure). The term *comorbidity* is therefore used to distinguish the main disease, that is, the one that causes dominant symptoms or requires the intervention by clinicians, from the concomitant, and sometimes incidental, diseases. On the other hand, the term *multimorbidity* is commonly used to define the coexistence of 2 or more diseases in the same individual that are thought to negatively influence each other. Multimorbidity is common in people in advanced ages; often, the terms *comorbidity* and *multimorbidity* are used indistinguishably. An interesting perspective comes from the theory of network medicine,[1] based on the idea that human diseases are not independent of each other but are the consequence of different biological processes that interact in a complex network, defined as *diseasome*. The clinical implication of this assumption is that the diseases should not be treated separately. For the purpose of the article, the term *comorbidity*

Disclosure Statement: The author declares he has no commercial or financial conflicts of interest related to the topic.
Dipartimento di Biomedicina e Medicina Specialistica, Sezione di Pneumologia, University of Palermo, Via Trabucco 180, Palermo 90146, Italy
E-mail address: nicola.scichilone@unipa.it

will be used to identify the conditions that may occur in the elderly respiratory patient. In addition, only chronic noncommunicable respiratory diseases, such as asthma, chronic obstructive pulmonary disease (COPD), and idiopathic lung fibrosis, will be discussed.

Most older respiratory patients have multiple coexisting conditions; indeed, more than 50% of older adults have 3 or more chronic conditions. However, recommendations on management of respiratory diseases are based on studies with restrictive inclusion criteria and thus subjects that are not representative of general population.[2]

The coexistence of multiple illnesses in the elderly patient is mainly owing to the association between increasing aging and incidence of chronic diseases and the development of complications of existing diseases over time. In this scenario, the presence of comorbidities is considered the norm in the most advanced ages and contributes to the complexity of disease. Indeed, the management of respiratory disease in the elderly becomes a challenge for clinicians in daily practice, as they have to take into account the interaction of respiratory with nonrespiratory illnesses. In this context, comorbidities should be treated appropriately and independently of the underlying respiratory disease, and multidisciplinary management should be part of routine assessment.

ASTHMA

Comorbidities are an important driver of asthma-related costs.[3] It is well accepted that the occurrence of comorbidities influences quality of life of older asthmatics,[4] and it is therefore plausible to hypothesize that comorbidities may account for poorer asthma outcomes in this population. Most importantly, deaths from asthma or nonrespiratory diseases mostly occur in older individuals,[5] and comorbid conditions may play a role in this regard. Depression[6] and atrial fibrillation,[7] in particular, affect asthma treatment outcomes in the elderly.

Asthma treatment is often based on inhaled medications: problems with the use of inhaler devices are common in the elderly and can, in turn, affect the level of adherence to treatment. For instance, a strong relationship between impairment of cognitive function and the inability to properly use the inhaler has been shown.[8] Depression is strongly related to poor asthma control and quality of life in the elderly.[6] In addition, anxiety and depression are related with overperception or underperception of asthma symptoms, and this may cause a misclassification of asthma severity.[9] Based on these observations, mood status should be routinely investigated. Different questionnaires are available to evaluate mood changes in the elderly, including the Geriatric Depression Scale and the Hospital Anxiety and Depression Scale.

Recently, atrial fibrillation has been associated with asthma,[7] suggesting that asthma may initiate atrial fibrillation, most probably because of β-agonists treatment. Moreover, the use of systemic and inhaled corticosteroids and bronchodilators seems to be linked to increased risk of atrial fibrillation in elderly individuals with asthma; on the other hand, medications often used by elderly patients, like ß-adrenergic blockers, may elicit or worsen bronchoconstriction. Soriano and colleagues[10] reported an increased risk of myocardial infarction and angina in asthmatic patients. Interestingly, the metabolic syndrome could be linked to asthma by sharing a common inflammatory pattern as suggested by Scichilone and colleagues[11] and by Barochia and colleagues.[12] Specifically, small low-density lipoproteins could lead to the amplification of the inflammatory cascade in asthma. COPD is an important comorbidity of asthma, and the prevalence of overlap between these 2 diseases increases with age.[10] A novel nosologic entity has been described, namely, the asthma-COPD overlap syndrome.

Patients with this syndrome have been found to have worse quality of life and increased mortality compared with age-matched asthmatics.[13]

The association between asthma and cataracts is of particular relevance in the elderly, given the high prevalence of cataracts in this population. Inhaled corticosteroids[14] are hypothesized to play a role in inducing cataracts; however, the risk of cataract development with inhaled corticosteroids is low,[15] and data on this relationship are inconsistent.[16] On the other hand, a significant increase in cataracts has been seen with the use of oral corticosteroids.[17] Hyperglycemia may develop in asthmatics as a result of the long-term use of systemic corticosteroids, and this is exacerbated in older subjects who already suffer from this condition. Similarly, osteoporosis is common in the elderly and may be complicated by the use of corticosteroids. Indeed, asthma has been recognized as a risk factor for osteoporotic fractures in the older patients.[18] To date, a clear distinction between the detrimental effects of inhaled and systemic corticosteroids has not been made.

CHRONIC OBSTRUCTIVE PULMONARY DISEASE

In the 2010 GOLD (Global Initiative for Chronic Obstructive Lung Disease) edition,[19] comorbidities were classified as coincidental, intercurrent, sharing common pathways, and complicating. Overall, this concept could be applied to other chronic respiratory diseases. Coincidental comorbidities are coexisting chronic conditions with unrelated pathogenesis, whose prevalence increases with aging and may complicate the management of COPD. This is the case in bowel or prostate cancer, depression, diabetes mellitus, Parkinson disease, dementia, and arthritis. Intercurrent comorbidities are represented by acute illnesses, such as upper respiratory tract infections, which may have a more severe impact in patients with chronic disease or may require different treatment. Comorbidities with common pathophysiology are other smoking-related diseases such as ischemic heart disease and lung cancer. Finally, complicating diseases are those that affect the management of COPD (eg, gastroesophageal reflux disease), both in terms of disease-to-disease interaction and drug-to-drug interaction.

Agusti and colleagues[20] proposed the systemic inflammome, which may account for higher rates of all-cause mortality in COPD. The prevalence of comorbidities in patients with COPD was assessed by Divo and collaborators[21] who identified comorbidities significantly associated with increased mortality (comorbidome). However, Vanfleteren and colleagues[22] did not find any association between comorbidities and mortality. Interestingly, Agusti and colleagues[23] proposed a model of vascularly interconnected diseases in which the lung is the source of signals that induce the inflammatory responses.

LUNG FIBROSIS

Idiopathic pulmonary fibrosis is a severe, progressive disease with poor prognosis at the time of diagnosis.[24] In subjects with idiopathic pulmonary fibrosis, comorbidities are common and mainly characterized by gastroesophageal reflux,[25] pulmonary hypertension,[26] and COPD.[27] In a systematic review, Raghu and colleagues[28] concluded that COPD, pulmonary hypertension, and obstructive sleep apnea are common in most study populations, although to various extents. Because systemic corticosteroids have been the main treatment of idiopathic pulmonary fibrosis, they may have contributed to the high prevalence of diabetes mellitus in this population. Mortality is associated with the coexistence of COPD and pulmonary hypertension.[28]

PHARMACOLOGIC TREATMENT

The pharmacologic treatment of chronic lung diseases in the elderly is extrapolated from evidence based on treatment of younger populations. This extrapolation can be made because older age has always been an exclusion criterion for eligibility for randomized clinical trials. In addition, comorbidities account for most recruitment failures, thus leading to the discrepancy between real life patients and experimental study populations. Scichilone and colleagues[29] and Battaglia and colleagues[2] recently showed that COPD and asthmatic patients enrolled in randomized clinical trials are not fully representative of patients encountered in clinical practice. There is a clear need for randomized clinical trials that include the elderly with the aim of expanding knowledge on pharmacologic treatment of respiratory diseases in these individuals. Furthermore, comorbidities are associated with polypharmacotherapy, which in turn is among the most important risk factors for adverse drug reactions in the elderly.[30] Comorbidities can influence the absorption, distribution, metabolism, and excretion of respiratory drugs. In addition, pharmacokinetics and pharmacodynamics of the respiratory drugs may be influenced by the drug-to-drug and the drug-to-disease interactions. If these aspects are not properly addressed in clinical practice, the likelihood that treatment failure or side effects occur increases.

Among potential side effects of inhaled corticosteroids, cataracts and osteoporosis are of particular interest, as they represent frequent comorbidities in the elderly population, perhaps associated with long-term oral corticosteroid use. Long acting β2-adrenergics–associated side effects are rare and of modest clinical importance, including muscular tremors and tachycardia. β2-agonists induce a net influx of intravascular potassium into cells. Thus, in older patients, hypokalemia, QT prolongation, tachycardia and tremor, which are mediated by the systemic drug absorption and are dose dependent, become serious adverse effects. Of course, the coexistence of cardiovascular disorders increases the frequency and severity of side effects.[31] Anticholinergics may induce urinary hesitancy, constipation, and exacerbations of glaucoma, all of which would be significant in elderly patients. The most frequent side effects are dry mouth and unpleasant taste, contributing in older people to reduced ability to speak, mucosal damage, and respiratory infection because of the reduction of antimicrobial activity of saliva. *Theophylline* may cause cardiovascular side effects such as supraventricular tachycardia and arrhythmias including potentially fatal events like ventricular arrhythmias. The side-effect profile of this drug, interactions with other medications, and need to monitor blood levels limit its use in the elderly. One therapeutic option for elderly patients with severe allergic asthma is anti-IgE therapy with the monoclonal antibody omalizumab. Potential adverse effects of anti-IgE therapy include an increased risk of parasitic infection, which should be properly addressed in those of advanced age.[32] There is still lack of data on safety of other biologic drugs, such as mepolizumab, in real life settings.

In addition to affecting pharmacologic treatment, comorbidities may impair the ability to use inhalation devices[33]; for example, arthritis of hands and fingers causes hand grip problems, visual or cognitive impairments affect the ability to properly use the inhaled device, and anxiety and depression can reduce the adherence to treatment. It follows that the choice of the proper inhaler should also take into account the relative contribution of concomitant diseases and the patient's physical and mental limitations.

Multidimensional Assessment

Chronic respiratory diseases in the elderly cannot be adequately managed without taking into account the complexity of the interaction with comorbid conditions. This

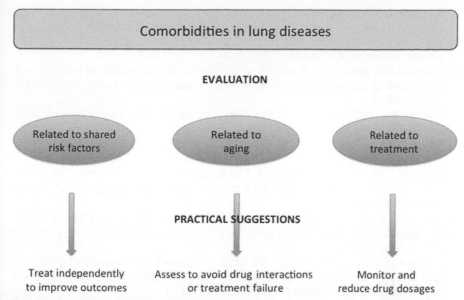

Fig. 1. Evaluation and practical suggestions for the assessment of comorbidities in clinical practice.

assumption implies a multidimensional assessment, which identifies priorities and strategies in the management of older respiratory patients. Some screening tools, such as the Mini-Mental State Examination and the clock drawing tests, should be routinely used in the elderly population. Indeed, they can predict the inability to perform spirometry.[34] Evaluation of walking speed should also be included in multidimensional assessment protocols. Different methods for gait speed evaluation are available, all of which predict mortality.[35] In patients with respiratory diseases, the 6-minute walk test seems preferable because it allows the detection of functional limitations.

SUMMARY

Noncommunicable chronic respiratory diseases are associated with aging and are often accompanied by comorbidities. The management of chronic respiratory diseases in the elderly therefore requires a comprehensive strategy. **Fig. 1** suggests a practical approach to the proper assessment of comorbidities. Unfortunately, older age frequently represents an exclusion criterion for eligibility in clinical trials, and current respiratory medications have rarely been tested in elderly populations. Absorption, distribution, metabolism, and excretion of respiratory drugs can be variably affected by age-associated comorbidities. Similarly, the drug-to-drug interactions may reduce the effectiveness of the inhaled medications and increase the risk of side effects. For these reasons, multidimensional management becomes mandatory in chronic respiratory patients of advanced age.

REFERENCES

1. Barabasi AL, Gulbahce N, Loscalzo J. Network medicine: a network-based approach to human disease. Nat Rev Genet 2011;12(1):56–68.

2. Battaglia S, Basile M, Spatafora M, et al. Are asthmatics enrolled in randomized trials representative of real-life outpatients? Respiration 2015;89(5):383–9.

3. Bahadori K, Doyle-Waters MM, Marra C, et al. Economic burden of asthma: a systematic review. BMC Pulm Med 2009;9:24.

4. Campos MA, Alazemi S, Zhang G, et al. Clinical characteristics of subjects with symptoms of alpha1-antitrypsin deficiency older than 60 years. Chest 2009; 135(3):600–8.

5. Gibson PG, McDonald VM, Marks GB. Asthma in older adults. Lancet 2010; 376(9743):803–13.

6. Krauskopf KA, Sofianou A, Goel MS, et al. Depressive symptoms, low adherence, and poor asthma outcomes in the elderly. J Asthma 2013;50(3):260–6.

7. Chan WL, Yang KP, Chao TF, et al. The association of asthma and atrial fibrillation–a nationwide population-based nested case-control study. Int J Cardiol 2014;176(2):464–9.

8. Allen SC, Jain M, Ragab S, et al. Acquisition and short-term retention of inhaler techniques require intact executive function in elderly subjects. Age Ageing 2003;32(3):299–302.

9. Steele AM, Meuret AE, Millard MW, et al. Discrepancies between lung function and asthma control: asthma perception and association with demographics and anxiety. Allergy Asthma Proc 2012;33(6):500–7.

10. Soriano JB, Visick GT, Muellerova H, et al. Patterns of comorbidities in newly diagnosed COPD and asthma in primary care. Chest 2005;128(4):2099–107.

11. Scichilone N, Rizzo M, Benfante A, et al. Serum low density lipoprotein subclasses in asthma. Respir Med 2013;107(12):1866–72.

12. Barochia AV, Kaler M, Cuento RA, et al. Serum apolipoprotein A-I and large high-density lipoprotein particles are positively correlated with FEV1 in atopic asthma. Am J Respir Crit Care Med 2015;191(9):990–1000.

13. Sorino C, Pedone C, Scichilone N. Fifteen-year mortality of patients with asthma-COPD overlap syndrome. Eur J Intern Med 2016;34:72–7.

14. Battaglia S, Cardillo I, Lavorini F, et al. Safety considerations of inhaled corticosteroids in the elderly. Drugs Aging 2014;31(11):787–96.

15. Jick SS, Vasilakis-Scaramozza C, Maier WC. The risk of cataract among users of inhaled steroids. Epidemiology 2001;12(2):229–34.

16. Mattishent K, Thavarajah M, Blanco P, et al. Meta-review: adverse effects of inhaled corticosteroids relevant to older patients. Drugs 2014;74(5):539–47.

17. Walsh LJ, Wong CA, Oborne J, et al. Adverse effects of oral corticosteroids in relation to dose in patients with lung disease. Thorax 2001;56(4):279–84.

18. Dam TT, Harrison S, Fink HA, et al, Osteoporotic Fractures in Men (MrOS) Research Group. Bone mineral density and fractures in older men with chronic obstructive pulmonary disease or asthma. Osteoporos Int 2010;21(8):1341–9.

19. Global Initiative for Chronic Obstructive Lung Disease (GOLD): Global strategy for the diagnosis, management and prevention of COPD. 2010. Available at: http://www.goldcopd.org/. Accessed January 10, 2017.

20. Agusti A, Edwards LD, Rennard SI, et al. Persistent systemic inflammation is associated with poor clinical outcomes in COPD: a novel phenotype. PLoS One 2012;7(5):e37483.

21. Divo M, Cote C, de Torres JP, et al. Comorbidities and risk of mortality in patients with chronic obstructive pulmonary disease. Am J Respir Crit Care Med 2012; 186(2):155–61.

22. Vanfleteren LE, Spruit MA, Groenen M, et al. Clusters of comorbidities based on validated objective measurements and systemic inflammation in patients with

chronic obstructive pulmonary disease. Am J Respir Crit Care Med 2013;187(7): 728–35.

23. Agusti A, Barbera JA, Wouters EF, et al. Lungs, bone marrow, and adipose tissue. A network approach to the pathobiology of chronic obstructive pulmonary disease. Am J Respir Crit Care Med 2013;188(12):1396–406.

24. Raghu G, Collard HR, Egan JJ, et al. An official ATS/ERS/JRS/ALAT statement: idiopathic pulmonary fibrosis: evidence-based guidelines for diagnosis and management. Am J Respir Crit Care Med 2011;183(6):788–824.

25. Raghu G, Freudenberger TD, Yang S, et al. High prevalence of abnormal acid gastro-oesophageal reflux in idiopathic pulmonary fibrosis. Eur Respir J 2006; 27(1):136–42.

26. Nadrous HF, Pellikka PA, Krowka MJ, et al. Pulmonary hypertension in patients with idiopathic pulmonary fibrosis. Chest 2005;128(4):2393–9.

27. Mejia M, Carrillo G, Rojas-Serrano J, et al. Idiopathic pulmonary fibrosis and emphysema: decreased survival associated with severe pulmonary arterial hypertension. Chest 2009;136(1):10–5.

28. Raghu G, Amatto VC, Behr J, et al. Comorbidities in idiopathic pulmonary fibrosis patients: a systematic literature review. Eur Respir J 2015;46(4):1113–30.

29. Scichilone N, Basile M, Battaglia S, et al. What proportion of chronic obstructive pulmonary disease outpatients is eligible for inclusion in randomized clinical trials? Respiration 2014;87(1):11–7.

30. Onder G, Petrovic M, Tangiisuran B, et al. Development and validation of a score to assess risk of adverse drug reactions among in-hospital patients 65 years or older: the GerontoNet ADR risk score. Arch Intern Med 2010;170(13):1142–8.

31. Centanni S, Carlucci P, Santus P, et al. Non-pulmonary effects induced by the addition of formoterol to budesonide therapy in patients with mild or moderate persistent asthma. Respiration 2000;67(1):60–4.

32. Verma P, Randhawa I, Klaustermeyer WB. Clinical efficacy of omalizumab in an elderly veteran population with severe asthma. Allergy Asthma Proc 2011; 32(5):346–50.

33. Hanania NA, Sharma G, Sharafkhaneh A. COPD in the elderly patient. Semin Respir Crit Care Med 2010;31(5):596–606.

34. Allen SC, Baxter M. A comparison of four tests of cognition as predictors of inability to perform spirometry in old age. Age Ageing 2009;38(5):537–41.

35. Studenski S, Perera S, Patel K, et al. Gait speed and survival in older adults. JAMA 2011;305(1):50–8.

UNITED STATES POSTAL SERVICE® — Statement of Ownership, Management, and Circulation (All Periodicals Publications Except Requester Publications)

1. Publication Title	2. Publication Number	3. Filing Date
CLINICS IN GERIATRIC MEDICINE	000 – 704	9/13/2017

4. Issue Frequency	5. Number of Issues Published Annually	6. Annual Subscription Price
FEB, MAY, AUG, NOV	4	$273.00

7. Complete Mailing Address of Known Office of Publication (Not printer) (Street, city, county, state, and ZIP+4®)

ELSEVIER INC.
230 Park Avenue, Suite 800
New York, NY 10169

Contact Person
STEPHEN R. BUSHING
Telephone (Include area code)
215-239-3688

8. Complete Mailing Address of Headquarters or General Business Office of Publisher (Not printer)

ELSEVIER INC.
230 Park Avenue, Suite 800
New York, NY 10169

9. Full Names and Complete Mailing Addresses of Publisher, Editor, and Managing Editor (Do not leave blank)

Publisher (Name and complete mailing address)
ADRIANNE BRIGIDO, ELSEVIER INC.
1600 JOHN F KENNEDY BLVD. SUITE 1800
PHILADELPHIA, PA 19103-2899

Editor (Name and complete mailing address)
JESSICA MCCOOL, ELSEVIER INC.
1600 JOHN F KENNEDY BLVD. SUITE 1800
PHILADELPHIA, PA 19103-2899

Managing Editor (Name and complete mailing address)
PATRICK MANLEY, ELSEVIER INC.
1600 JOHN F KENNEDY BLVD. SUITE 1800
PHILADELPHIA, PA 19103-2899

10. Owner (Do not leave blank. If the publication is owned by a corporation, give the name and address of the corporation immediately followed by the names and addresses of all stockholders owning or holding 1 percent or more of the total amount of stock. If not owned by a corporation, give the names and addresses of the individual owners. If owned by a partnership or other unincorporated firm, give its name and address as well as those of each individual owner. If the publication is published by a nonprofit organization, give its name and address.)

Full Name	Complete Mailing Address
WHOLLY OWNED SUBSIDIARY OF REED/ELSEVIER, US HOLDINGS	1600 JOHN F KENNEDY BLVD. SUITE 1800 PHILADELPHIA, PA 19103-2899

11. Known Bondholders, Mortgagees, and Other Security Holders Owning or Holding 1 Percent or More of Total Amount of Bonds, Mortgages, or Other Securities. If none, check box ☒ None

Full Name	Complete Mailing Address
N/A	

12. Tax Status (For completion by nonprofit organizations authorized to mail at nonprofit rates) (Check one)
The purpose, function, and nonprofit status of this organization and the exempt status for federal income tax purposes:
☒ Has Not Changed During Preceding 12 Months
☐ Has Changed During Preceding 12 Months (Publisher must submit explanation of change with this statement)

13. Publication Title
CLINICS IN GERIATRIC MEDICINE

14. Issue Date for Circulation Data Below
MAY 2017

15. Extent and Nature of Circulation			Average No. Copies Each Issue During Preceding 12 Months	No. Copies of Single Issue Published Nearest to Filing Date
a. Total Number of Copies (Net press run)			298	212
b. Paid Circulation (By Mail and Outside the Mail)	(1)	Mailed Outside-County Paid Subscriptions Stated on PS Form 3541 (Include paid distribution above nominal rate, advertiser's proof copies, and exchange copies)	110	94
	(2)	Mailed In-County Paid Subscriptions Stated on PS Form 3541 (Include paid distribution above nominal rate, advertiser's proof copies, and exchange copies)	0	0
	(3)	Paid Distribution Outside the Mails Including Sales Through Dealers and Carriers, Street Vendors, Counter Sales, and Other Paid Distribution Outside USPS®	69	57
	(4)	Paid Distribution by Other Classes of Mail Through the USPS (e.g., First-Class Mail®)	0	0
c. Total Paid Distribution (Sum of 15b (1), (2), (3), and (4))			179	151
d. Free or Nominal Rate Distribution (By Mail and Outside the Mail)	(1)	Free or Nominal Rate Outside-County Copies included on PS Form 3541	65	61
	(2)	Free or Nominal Rate In-County Copies Included on PS Form 3541	0	0
	(3)	Free or Nominal Rate Copies Mailed at Other Classes Through the USPS (e.g., First-Class Mail)	0	0
	(4)	Free or Nominal Rate Distribution Outside the Mail (Carriers or other means)	65	61
e. Total Free or Nominal Rate Distribution (Sum of 15d (1), (2), (3) and (4))			65	61
f. Total Distribution (Sum of 15c and 15e)			244	212
g. Copies not Distributed (See Instructions to Publishers #4 (page #3))			54	0
h. Total (Sum of 15f and g)			298	212
i. Percent Paid (15c divided by 15f times 100)			73.36%	71.23%

* If you are claiming electronic copies, go to line 16 on page 3. If you are not claiming electronic copies, skip to line 17 on page 3.

16. Electronic Copy Circulation	Average No. Copies Each Issue During Preceding 12 Months	No. Copies of Single Issue Published Nearest to Filing Date
a. Paid Electronic Copies ▲	0	0
b. Total Paid Print Copies (Line 15c) + Paid Electronic Copies (Line 16a) ▲	179	151
c. Total Print Distribution (Line 15f) + Paid Electronic Copies (Line 16a) ▲	244	212
d. Percent Paid (Both Print & Electronic Copies) (16b divided by 16c × 100) ▲	73.36%	71.23%

☒ I certify that 50% of all my distributed copies (electronic and print) are paid above a nominal price.

17. Publication of Statement of Ownership
☒ If the publication is a general publication, publication of this statement is required. Will be printed in the NOVEMBER 2017 issue of this publication. ☐ Publication not required.

18. Signature and Title of Editor, Publisher, Business Manager, or Owner

STEPHEN R. BUSHING - INVENTORY DISTRIBUTION CONTROL MANAGER

Date 9/18/2017

I certify that all information furnished on this form is true and complete. I understand that anyone who furnishes false or misleading information on this form or who omits material or information requested on the form may be subject to criminal sanctions (including fines and imprisonment) and/or civil sanctions (including civil penalties).

Moving?

Make sure your subscription moves with you!

To notify us of your new address, find your **Clinics Account Number** (located on your mailing label above your name), and contact customer service at:

Email: journalscustomerservice-usa@elsevier.com

800-654-2452 (subscribers in the U.S. & Canada)
314-447-8871 (subscribers outside of the U.S. & Canada)

Fax number: 314-447-8029

Elsevier Health Sciences Division
Subscription Customer Service
3251 Riverport Lane
Maryland Heights, MO 63043

*To ensure uninterrupted delivery of your subscription, please notify us at least 4 weeks in advance of move.

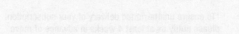

Printed and bound by CPI Group (UK) Ltd, Croydon, CR0 4YY

07/10/2024

01040504-0012